AUTHENTICITY
IN
NURSING

This is an IndieMosh book
brought to you by MoshPit Publishing
an imprint of Mosher's Business Support Pty Ltd
PO Box 4363
Penrith NSW 2750
indiemosh.com.au

Copyright © Pete Smith 2021
belowtenthousand.com

The moral right of the author has been asserted in accordance with the Copyright Amendment (Moral Rights) Act 2000.

All rights reserved. Except as permitted under the Australian Copyright Act 1968 (for example, fair dealing for the purposes of study, research, criticism or review) no part of this publication may be reproduced, stored in a retrieval system, or transmitted in any form or by any means, electronic, mechanical, photocopying, recording or otherwise, without the written permission of the publisher.

Cataloguing-in-Publication entry is available from the National Library of Australia: http://catalogue.nla.gov.au/

Title: Authenticity in Nursing

Subtitle: Fit for purpose

Author: Smith, Pete (1963–)

ISBNs: 978-1-922542-20-5 (paperback)
978-1-922542-21-2 (ebook – epub)
978-1-922542-22-9 (ebook – mobi)

Subjects: MEDICAL: Ethics; Nursing / Social, Ethical & Legal Issues; Nursing / Management & Leadership; Nursing / Nurse & Patient

The author has made every effort to ensure that the information in this book was correct at the time of publication. However, the author and publisher accept no liability for any loss, damage or disruption incurred by the reader or any other person arising from any action taken or not taken based on the content of this book. The author recommends seeking third party advice and considering all options prior to making any decision or taking action in regard to the content of this book.

Cover design and layout by Ally Mosher at allymosher.com

Kimguard fabric image from Adobe Stock.

AUTHENTICITY
IN
NURSING

Fit for purpose

PETE SMITH

Also by Pete Smith:

THE BELOW TEN THOUSAND WAY

to a clinician-led safety culture

belowtenthousand.com

Introduction

If your name was Johann Sebastian Bach and you wanted to write a concerto, the story your music would tell is a journey of self-discovery.

That journey would include a journeying out, the unearthing of your individual Authenticity, and a prodigal journey home.

Bach's concertos are infused with the timeless narratives of antiquity, and what makes them great is the fact that each and every one of them is our own story, the story of a person, the story of a life, the story of self-forgiveness and the story of how each and every one of us can find meaning within the seemingly chaotic vicissitudes of life.

Nursing is an art as well as a science.

It is a calling to those fascinated by the humanity incumbent in life.

Amidst the all-encompassing investment of soul and sacrifice that is required in order to tend to others needs, a single thread shines through—a thread of Authenticity that strives for recognition, a shining strand of light that tethers us to our duty of care and guides our actions throughout our careers.

It is not an easy thing, to be a nurse.

And yet, despite the difficulties stacked against us, we return each day to give all we can, and then give some more.

We go beyond, simply because it is asked of us.

We also succumb, each day, to the recklessness of a system which prides itself on the delivery of safe care despite the evidence that, at present, safe care is a mirage, a mass delusion, an idiotic figment of our grandiose imagination.

Nurses' Authenticity is challenged at every turn because nurses lack positional power and a voice, despite being the core deliverers of frontline care.

For nurses, the journey out is one of despair.

The recapitulation is the finding of the inner voice, the discovery of that inner Authenticity that empowers us to stand in the face of the onslaught and advocate for our patients and ourselves.

The long and winding journey home is no less perilous, and no less demanding.

In the end, the idea of 'home' is that we become a beacon of understanding, a lighthouse resolute in the surge of the storm, an understanding that we, as angels with broken wings, stand alone as fragile links in a tenuous human chain to offer a therapeutic balm of humanity to a ceaseless tide of human suffering that bursts in waves upon our shore.

That we strive with Authenticity is what makes us strong.

That we strive with Authenticity is what makes us tenacious in our delivery of excellent care.

That we are compassionate in our Authenticity is what makes us humble.

The greatest concerto of our lives is the conduct of our journey.

The crescendo is the celebration of becoming a beacon of hope on life's shore.

The storm shall pass, the sun shall shine, and a settled ocean of clinician and patient safety, as simple as it is, will lap placidly at our feet, the only sound the quietude of listening and the gentle splash of realistic expectation.

In Authenticity, the nurse finds a deep calm and a deeper knowledge of the orchestra of life.

Dedication

I don't know if it is a fair thing to do, to plunge someone back into a treasure chest of painful memories.

But I think I'm going to do it anyway.

Whilst Jasmine's Mum is fatigued, exhausted by her desperate effort to induce meaningful change in healthcare, Jasmine remains forever her energetic, funny and at times fiery toddler.

And will eternally do so.

Her life stolen at twenty months, the passage of time will not weary little Jasmine.

But for Joanne, Jasmine's mum, the memory of her beautiful baby girl, the light of her life, will remain on hold forever.

Every 15th of February Joanne will relive the moment of Jasmine's passing in every stark detail.

All Joanne wants is for healthcare professionals to learn the lessons there to be learned from Jasmine's death so that no one else must suffer the agonies she has been forced to endure.

Deep learning is not something we as healthcare professionals are keen to do.

Sure we learn all the time.

New drugs, new techniques, new equipment.

But ...

Still the same old healthcare system, too scared to look inside of itself for fear of what it may find.

On a journey to ... it can never be 'healing', because how can you 'heal' from a black hole gaping at the centre of the universe of your soul?—Joanne has demonstrated her truly incredible Authenticity.

The system that quelled the life spirit of her baby girl has not.

As I continue to write my book on Authenticity in nursing, I always imagined I would dedicate it to John Gibbs and Rob Tomlinson, two of the most Authentic nurses I know.

But I'm going to have to apologise to them.

Sorry guys. You are going to have to wait.

Book Two belongs to someone else:

To Jasmine and Joanne,
A most angelic memory,
And a most Authentic struggle to be heard.

Pete

http://www.mothersinstinct.co.uk/patient-stories

Rules of Engagement

Assume, in the first instance,
That nothing I say is true.
Then, stop
Take a look around
And see what you see.

(Pete Smith, 2021)

Authentic, a Definition

According to Merriam-Webster, an acceptable definition of the word 'Authentic' is as follows:

Authentic:

- worthy of acceptance or belief as conforming to or based on fact
- conforming to an original so as to reproduce essential features
- made or done the same way as an original
- not false or imitation: REAL, ACTUAL.

Authenticity as a concept is of particular interest in psychology. It also arises as a topic for contemplation in existential philosophy and aesthetics.

Wikipedia states: "In existentialism, Authenticity is the degree to which an individual's actions are congruent with their beliefs and desires, despite external pressures."

Authenticity is a complex topic.

In a dynamic, ever-changing world, the contemporary evolves from the classic.

The pressure to conform to the rigours of society is culturally nuanced and in conflict with the pressure to conform to one's own beliefs, values and desires.

Conflict therefore creates a dynamic tension arising from these internal and external, often combative, sources.

Authenticity has an aesthetic quality.

Integrity is the behavioural expression of that Authenticity.

Words can lie.

It is behaviour that tells the truth.

Contents

Also by Pete Smith: iv

Introduction v

Dedication viii

Rules of Engagement x

Authentic, a Definition xi

Samaritans, Each and Every One 1

A Midwinter Morning Dream 4

Waking Up to Contentment 7

Know Thyself 9

Trend Setting 13

Will 15

Game Theory of Burnout 19

High Effort or Low Effort? 21

Surgery Stat! 25

Malicious Compliance 28

Dead Man's Anchor 30

Soil 32

Therapeutic Window 34

Microclimates 36

The 1.5 Metre Rule 38

The Fractal Nature of Circles of Influence.................. 40

Integration of a Safety Culture 44

The Bully Bell... 46

White Cow 51

Top Down... 55

Crabs.. 58

Cognitive Laboratory... 59

Mission Brown 64

Red Flags 66

So How do Red Flags Help? 69

The Authenticity of Standards 71

The Plimsoll Line 74

Self-care... 76

Bricks and Mortarboards 79

Tragedy of the Commons... 81

Max 86

Faster, Faster Too Busy to Care 88

"I will stuff their mouths with gold" 91

Enabling Advocacy 94

Learning with Purpose 99

READD 100

Timelessness in the Desert 115

Human Factors 118

Regenerating a Supportive Culture 120

Exam question 126

About the Author 127

Samaritans, Each and Every One

The only question I remember in my hospital interview to become a nurse was pitched to me by the then Director of Nursing at Grafton Base Hospital, Matron Higham:

"Why do you want to become a nurse?"

"I don't know," was my naive reply, though I had done other things and failed at them all, and I thought nursing might be something I might be good at.

How I got an offer to commence Preliminary Training School I don't know.

In retrospect, I can only thank Matron Higham for the trajectory she set me upon because, in part, of the simply incredibly amazing people I have had the good fortune to have been surrounded by all my nursing life.

A career in helping people should be the most noble, enabling and affirming life one could have.

A career in nursing should be a crown jewel in the spiritual journey of living of a well-lived life.

So it interests me as to why nursing, whilst uplifting to many, also has the potential to destroy unceremoniously some whose only crime is to try their best to live up to their own, and society's, expectations in the simple endeavour to care for those in need.

The Good Samaritan of biblical fame lost little in attending to the needs of the philistine.

Nurses, each and every one, on the other hand, are the epicentre of a maelstrom of collateral damage suffered, first by themselves and then, as second victims, their families and loved ones.

My belief is that the construct of the nursing identity is that of a healer. Through a long legacy of the artful application of rigorously tested science, the role of a nurse is simply to ease suffering.

It is a simple pretext which covers all aspects of physiology, psychology and existential fear:

To ease suffering, and, where possible, to heal.

To any nurse, the image of Florence Nightingale is burned into their brain.

It forms a permanent imprint upon our amygdala, whether we want it or not, like it or not, rail against it or not.

As usual, the cultural image of the lady with the lamp is different from the actual DNA- and emotion-clad personage.

The truth is different in a thousand little ways from the legend, but it is the 'legend' which has supplanted the 'real' in our minds.

As an aesthetic construct, the 'idea' of Florence is what we subscribe to. The rest becomes mere hearsay.

It is with this construct that we create the beliefs and values we ascertain as 'Authentic' in our field.

It is against this construct that we measure ourselves.

There is a Florence in every nurse.

You can tell a nurse by their smile: the all-knowing, all-understanding smile of the compassionate person who has seen humanity in all its vast vulnerable nakedness and still chooses to put it all aside, give of themselves, and care.

So imagine the shock when nurses discover that their greatest virtue is used against them by a clandestine, intemperate society with a monopoly on misplaced self-interest.

Imagine the shock when a caring person finds the duty of care goes only one way.

Imagine the shock when a nurse discovers that they are expected to break their back for people who won't lift a finger to help themselves.

Imagine the shock when a nurse discovers that the culture of safety we so celebrate is in fact a crumbling ruin with little basis in fact.

What part of this is 'the Authentic'?

Can belief and fact find in us a truth?

A Midwinter Morning Dream

It was not a bad dream, as far as dreams go.

At an old farm at my mother's birthplace at Hernani, on a hairpin bend on a winding mountain road, stands the small old cottage of brown raw lumber flanked by the all-important frostbitten chimney.

I always imagine my mum as a small girl on this farm, standing stoic on the hill in the icy dawn, dress flapping in the wind, going about her traps to release the rabbits that would earn her the pittance that would fund her purchase of precious forever-loved books.

The cold mountain climate keeps the bracken fern thick and green down by the road where, almost obscured, first by the fact that it is so familiar, and second by the unkempt growth that surrounds it, stands a timeless old bus shelter with space for a huddle of just four small girls.

Beside it stands a memorial to Mary MacKillop, saint.

Just over the hill on former farming property, the roofs of industrial sheds have hastily grown at the first whiff of opportunity.

The sounds of timber mill saws can be heard drowning out the bellbirds, with their classic chime-like call.

It is familiar territory because I have dreamt of this place before.

What was strange for me was that the dream, so real, seemed so subconsciously linked to a problem I was grappling with, the problem of Authenticity.

In it there was a tribute to learning; the bus stop, quaint as it was, offering protection with the hope that knowledge would keep me safe.

The little altar, covered with moss, showed a saint in her humility, with the words "We are but trespassers here" etched underneath.

On the kerb was a new addition to the topography of my dream, the fire bell, gleaming, polished but, until that moment, unobserved.

I remember being glad that the warning system was right outside this house.

A few cars rushed close past on their way to the industrial estate, becoming airborne as they topped the crest on the gravel road, and that was it.

I woke up to a grey cat sleeping on my feet, a winter dawn sun peeping through the east window of the Chateau du Bunyip and the yodel of a magpie reminding me of its desire for breakfast.

The warning bell was the part of the dream that puzzled me.

In my dream, it was so perfectly in focus.

I wondered what role it was meant to play.

A warning about the book I was working on, that it was a warning to the healthcare profession that the

Authenticity of our lovingly nurtured past was in clear and present danger from system gone mad?

Or that it was a warning to me that I was on treacherous philosophic ground of which I had a paucity of understanding?

By appearance, the bell was still imminently functional, and its potential as a call for alarm was real.

It seemed the presence of the warning system meant that there were still opportunities to beat back the flames that would otherwise lead to our destruction.

It was an interesting dream that filled me more with hope than dread, albeit with a sense of confusion, and as I got on with my morning farming duties, the dream remained clear in my mind whilst my resoluteness remained calm in my heart.

It was time to claim my Authentic simple overgrown moral ancestral home, the aesthetic of which was perfect, exactly as it stood.

Waking Up to Contentment

If my dream was a metaphor for my idea of my own profession's Authenticity, it was a good one that I would happily own.

The idea of education was sound.

The idea of building competence on the shoulders of our ancestral greats was sound.

Even the notion of busy industry was sound because in productivity there is happiness.

To quote Mike and Michael from managertools.com, the claim that happy people are more productive is a fallacy.

In fact, they attest, the data shows the converse bears more truth: "Productive people become happy, and they become happy in their own right."

It is a nice little flip, because for a manager, trying to make people 'happy' is a thankless, bottomless pit.

Keeping them productive whilst still on the safe side of the 'Edge of Coping' is possible.

Workers, then, become responsible for their own contentment with life.

In other words, work done well is life affirming.

At Bunyip Creek we have a few rules.

One is, that each day we ask of ourselves:

- What shall we do?
- How shall we do it?
- When shall we stop?

The last question is the most important, and was crafted in the forge of my operating theatre clinical work.

'When shall we stop?' is the one question that keeps us most safe and effective in our work. and keeps the colours in life's rainbow.

It is the key to our contentment.

It is the one thing that keeps us Authentic in the pursuit of our strategic plan.

Know Thyself

The history of the search for the meaning of Authenticity goes back to the dawn of civilisation.

It is only when Homo sapiens clustered into social communities to benefit survival that we began the process of physically distancing ourselves from nature whilst never rising above our baboonish DNA.

The distancing from nature and the clustering into tribes spawned within us the spirit of domination.

Alpha behaviour, the will to dominate in itself, led to the challenge: "My word is Law."

Being brutish and summarily executable, it quickly overcame the notion of "My word is a contribution" that nature bestowed upon the gentler beta collaboratives.

To reconnect the 'Authenticity of the self' back to the those deprived of the right to their own individuality, maxims materialised.

The Oracle of Delphi preached moderation in all things and the fickleness of knowledge.

"Know thyself."

Socrates was proclaimed the wisest man in Athens, simply because Socrates knew he knew nothing.

Plato's Cave arose from Socrates influence and since that time, philosophers have tried to determine exactly what true Authenticity is, whilst psychologists have struggled to find ways that the individual may seek to 'behave' it.

It is Robert Sapolsky, a professor at Stanford University, who has taken us back the full circle in his study of stress in baboons.

Homo sapiens share 85% of baboon DNA, a commonality which is instructive.

Sapolsky travelled to Africa each year, closely observing the behaviour of a troupe of baboons and collecting data in his search for the origins of stress in primates.

What he found was astonishing.

First, he discovered that he hated baboons.

Baboons, he found, could collect all their nutritional requirements in just three hours every day.

Which meant that they could spend the other 21 hours of each day dreaming up ways to make the lives of their peers completely miserable.

With stunning precision.

Brutality and nastiness flowed one way—down the chain from the dominant members all the way to the bottom of the pecking order—in kicks, scratches, bites, theft and chases from alpha to beta to beyond.

So much for the notion of a baboon utopia!

As a baboon in the wild, your position on the social strata is a good predictor of your health and longevity.

The common link was stress hormones.

The alphas were the healthiest.

They had no stress because they were the originators of it.

They were the wind that made the waves that eventually crashed upon the rocks.

The second tier had stress, but once again were healthier because they knew exactly who they could kick, and how hard.

Like carriers of disease who show few clinical signs of the disease they possess but pass it on in full measure to those they infect, these baboons were carriers of stress.

Interestingly enough, research in the British Civil Service at around the same time unearthed exactly the same dynamics.

If you are interested, try watching the documentary *Stress: The Silent Killer*.

An incidental discovery led to an interesting finding.

The baboon troupe lived not too far from a resort and from time to time they raided the resort's rubbish heap.

Contaminated meat led to the deaths through botulism of a significant number of the troupe.

Devastated that years of research had been destroyed in a single moment, Sapolsky found other troupes and started his work all over again.

Years later he re-encountered his original troupe and discovered that something phenomenal had happened.

The troupe in its entirety was healthier than normal, and its members engaged in statistically significant increased supportive behaviours.

What had happened was interesting.

The baboons who had died were the first to the rubbish heap, the dominant, aggressive alpha baboons, and in one fell swoop, the highly competitive alphas had been eliminated from the troupe.

In their place rose, not new alphas, but a cohort of collaborative betas who then went on to maintain their social group, evicting newcomers bearing aggressive tendencies from their community, or teaching them to become more supportive.

In doing so, they were able to progress, longitudinally over time, a quantum shift in the culture of their community to the extent that benevolence, support and compassion ruled.

The moral to the story is that a more compassionate Authenticity is possible, but only if we place boundaries around the behaviours of those who would engage in sociopathy in order to gain advantage.

Please note: there is no need to kill anybody.

The secret is the *fortifying of realistic and concrete compassionate boundaries.*

Most of the history of human conquest has involved the attempt to achieve peace through expressions of psychological and behavioural brutality.

It is more Authentic, if we want peace, to gain peace through peaceful means.

Trend Setting

I'm down the paddock spraying weeds.

An invasive weed called fireweed (Senecio madagascariensis).

Left to its own devices it dominates pasture, overpowering the native grass species by its aggressive spread and its use of pheromones to suppress the germination of seeds of other species.

In short, it's a bully.

I realise, in my spraying, that what I am cognitively and biomechanically deferring to in my work is low-energy pattern identification based upon colour differentials, leaf structure and knowledge of mechanisms of spread.

Sapolsky's baboons fill the vacant spaces in my cognitive horizon.

The notion of early identification of sociopathic behaviour with the low effort low cost strategy of early elimination of dystopians enters my head.

After all, toxic patterns of behaviour do not arise overnight.

They are often identified well in advance of them becoming an end-stage problem.

For example, murderers such as Ivan Milat and the Anita Cobby killers were on the radar of police well before their heinous acts were committed, investigated and their guilt established.

In healthcare teams, the same could be said of sociopathic employees.

They come to us with an established pattern of toxic behaviour, and in our hustle to fill vacancies with anybody showing signs of life, we give them new pastures in which to spread their aggressive cheer.

Aggressive cheer, because sociopathic charm is what makes them stand out from the crowd.

In fireweed, it takes just eight days from flowering until the seed is set. Eight days before a million opportunities for spread occurs. Much germination occurs under the foliage radius, but some seeds gets spread by the wind across the paddock, creating new epicentres for invasion.

Toxicity begets toxicity.

One troupe of baboons learned to recognise the early signs of aggression and act to dispel it from their community.

As nurses working in a relentlessly high-pressure, high-risk clinical environment, it would be prudent if we were to learn to do the same.

As a manager, if my ONLY REAL JOB is to build my team, I'd want to make sure I was damned good at it.

Will

Authenticity is a tricky business. But it is only tricky if we think about it the wrong way.

As an example; in the nature or nurture debate, the difficulties arise only because we paint ourselves into a corner through an error in our thinking: by using the word 'or'.

The word 'or' sets up a dichotomy, whereas replacing it with the word 'and' sets up a responsibility to act.

To be Authentic to one's self seems on the surface to be a debate about 'will'.

To the uninitiated, it is easy to assume that if you are 'Authentic' then you will have sheer 'will' to you get what you think you deserve by any means necessary.

But that is so not true.

'Any means necessary' is a corruption of Authenticity, because in Authenticity, the means must justify the ends we aspire to.

On the flipside we also fail to consider that assuming our Authenticity means navigating and reconciling ourselves with our social contract.

To take an example, my old man at the time of writing is 90 years old. He drives an old Suzuki Stockman Ute which does 60 kph on the open road. He also crosses a busy road to get from one part of the property to another, an act he commits several times a day.

Where he chooses to cross, his vision is obscured by a very big, very old fig tree.

As part of his own Authenticity, he considers that he should retain the right to drive despite his declining psychomotor skills.

I would maintain that part of his social contract includes the fact that he doesn't have the right to kill someone driving innocently down a long straight at 100 kph by pulling out in front of them.

Yesterday a 20-year-old had to take significant evasive action to avoid colliding with the old man.

The lad came back and said to my father: "You nearly killed me!" To which the old man replied, "Well, you nearly killed me."

Ethics aside, free will, perceived rights, identity, social contract and Authenticity collide.

In the end, high Authenticity, whether of high free will or low free will, leads to peaceful benevolence.

Low Authenticity, whether of low free will or high free will, leads to angst.

The empirical difference between high and low Authenticity is the absence or presence of inner turmoil.

Gross inner turmoil leads to a struggle for identity, violence expressed internally or externally, and thus, suffering.

Inner calm leads to peace, and from peace, benevolence to self and others flows.

Back to nursing, the same mathematical function applies. Our social contract implies some conditions.

For example: 'First do no harm'; 'Treat everyone equally irrespective of race, creed, socioeconomics and behaviour'; 'Be competent'.

Because the identity of a nurse is tied up with these things, inner calm comes from our ability to reconcile our inner Authenticity with our externally imposed contract.

Where there is concordance, contentment reigns. Where there is divergence, angst arises.

As a nurse, therefore, every bit of our Authenticity, and thus our identity, hinges on our ability to practise with integrity in a timely, safe and effective way.

In other words, we aspire to a safety culture.

Where reality strikes discord into our ability to indulge in that safety culture, our Authenticity is challenged and our sense of identity becomes confused.

How important is it, therefore, to make participation in the safety culture a compulsory feature of our everyday work?

How important is it, then, to combat things that erode team trust, like bullying?

How important is it, then, to combat things that erode effective communication, like hierarchy, noise and distraction?

How important is it then, to combat things that erode work effectiveness, like poor systems processes and turbulent work flow?

How important is it, then, to combat things that erode psychomotor effectiveness, like fatigue and the overburden of miscalculated production pressure?

In short, the very identity of a nurse is at odds with almost every facet of modern-day healthcare provision, and because of this, the struggle to be Authentic becomes existentially all-consuming.

Game Theory of Burnout

Any day ever begins on a day like any other …

The world turns, the sun rises …

And yet …

Human emotion turns on a dime.

Game Theory is mathematics. It is the closest thing we have to a mathematical prediction of human behaviour.

"Mathematics?" you say.

And here I can feel your brain shutting down.

But maths isn't that hard. It's just numbers following simple rules. Where our heads explode is that simple rules can turn out to behave in quite complex ways.

So imagine this:

You have a choice of two jobs. One is on a factory floor making widgets. The other is nursing.

The first is mundane. The second you choose because you care.

Nursing is not a bad choice for the right person. Most people choose nursing because they want to help people.

There. That's not so bad, is it?

The next part is equally simple and nothing to do with you: Your employer gets to choose. High pay or low pay.

Simple.

The choices we make!

Meaningful work means you are meaningfully invested in the output of the work you are performing.

Because you are invested, you choose to work hard.

In fact, healthcare is generally regarded as meaningful work because nurses consider patient outcome and the easing of suffering important.

Nonmeaningful work means you couldn't care less whether the outcome is excellent or 'just good enough'. Even bad doesn't matter if you still get to turn up tomorrow, keep your job and not suffer any financial penalty.

Although people may find factory work nonmeaningful, it is a matter of beliefs and values as to whether it really is meaningless to you, or whether you find meaning in the delight of production, quality and community.

So what is important is the meaning you attach to your work.

High Effort or Low Effort?

Should you work hard or slacken off for the given amount of pay you receive for your work?

Working as a nurse, long hours, ridiculous workloads, circadian toxic rotating rosters, high cognitive, physical and emotional loads and poorly designed systems of work mean that, if you are meaningful invested in your work, you will do the seemingly impossible hard yards even though your pay is mediocre when benchmarked against similar professions.

In fact, Game Theory says that the probability of you saying "no" to any task asked of you is statistically low, especially if saying "no" means that some other person, a third party, someone you don't even know, will suffer.

The price of your compassion stacks negatively against positive utility payoffs such as how much pay you get at the end of each fortnight and the inner glow of doing good.

The total sum of your utility payoffs finishes up being low because of the cost of your increased effort, and in particular, the toll it takes on your physical and mental wellbeing, and that of your family.

The organisation, however, extracts a high fiscal value out of your meaningfully invested work.

At the point of burnout, the worker shifts from seeing work as meaningful to seeing work as nonmeaningful.

In nonmeaningful work the maximum utility payoff to the worker occurs when they choose to do as little as possible in order to keep their job.

The value of the burned-out employee to the employer descends to almost zero. Worse, the very identity of the nurse and her puzzled family lies in tatters.

It is a sad story that bears further examination.

Bad faith at work costs so much.

A lack of organisational compassion for the psycho-motor boundaries of human performance takes the nurse beyond the 'Edge of Coping'.

A lack of respect for the limits of time and infrastructure resources further extracts a toll which can only be paid by making nurses work harder, miss their breaks and stay beyond their scheduled time at the end of their shift.

The cumulative effect is that the nurse works to the point of exhaustion in an effort to prop up a non-sustainable system of work, when in fact, given what we know about Game Theory, the chance of the nurse saying "no" to any (even unreasonable) demand is functionally small.

Smart management would specify that in order to keep a nurse meaningfully invested in their crucial work, the prevention of harm or burnout would mean having systems in place that prevent the nurse from overcommitting.

Keeping nurses meaningfully invested in their work makes good business sense.

The payoff to the nurse is increased if the effort required is sustainable, and the organisation gets to keep their high payoff for the entirety of that nurse's career.

Appropriate staffing, hard boundaries which prevent fatigue, and good systems of work ensure that nurses stay meaningful, feel well and have energy for other facets of life, especially those that contribute positively to their own wellbeing.

Smash someone repeatedly, and what you get is pretty much what we get now in the healthcare system:

Clinicians, ordinary people who suffer high levels of burnout, high absenteeism, emotive conflict, errors in care, and suicide.

Sadly, the people we inflict these indignities upon are the ones who started out simply wanting to help others.

In the end, they can't even help themselves.

It is not their intelligence that lets them down. These people are without doubt bright.

It is the system itself and its lack of intelligent governance that dashes their hopes and offers no way out of the bind other than giving up and giving in.

Once you lose a clinician to nonmeaningful work, all profitability is lost. But that is the least of our problems.

Mortifyingly sad is the following statistic: In Geelong in one single year there were three junior doctor suicides.

What on earth happens when the best and brightest, three lives full of hope, find nothing but hopelessness in a job that SHOULD be the most empowering job of all—one filled with the joy of helping others in their time of need?

It might be called Game Theory, but it is not a game.

There are serious implications, but if system learning is lost to panic, if brutalising good people by insisting that they are tested to the point of destruction is the norm, then there is no hope.

Not for nurses.

Not for doctors.

Not for health executives.

Not for health economists.

Not for patients.

System failure is absolute, and it remains absolute because we fail to recognise system failure.

Is the opposite of Authenticity corruption?

Surgery Stat!

'Surgery Stat!' started life as an idea.

At the time I was the voluntary occupational health and safety representative for my theatres.

Early on in my time as a rep, I realised a simple flaw in our logic.

The Health and Safety Act is very specific in one thing:

Wherever the term 'health' is used in the Act, physical health and psychological health, by definition, are implied.

In my work, it was easy to identify where physical risks were involved.

What was impossible to achieve was respect for where psychological stressors were most prevalent, simply because psychological stress is more difficult to see.

Whenever I went to the front desk of theatres from where the supervisor managed the floor, I could see psychological harm.

Whenever I went into Recovery at peak times, I could see psychological harm.

Whenever I walked down the central corridor of theatres at 5:30 pm, I could see psychological harm.

Psychological harm was all around me, but it seemed that it so pervaded the environment of the operating theatre that no one paid it any attention.

What I saw was the stress of time pressure and how that time pressure infected every second of what we did so pervasively that it dominated our every thought.

There were a few toxic idiosyncrasies particular to our area.

One was that, although true emergencies happened at a frequency of about 5% of the time, we acted as though EVERYTHING was an emergency.

The second was that because we were so pressured for time, we acted as though we were busy ALL the time when in fact work intensity was often skewed in time, as though the illusion of busy-ness and the fact of busy-ness were both one and the same thing.

The third was that everything had to be done for everybody.

The operating theatre list, although it was grossly overbooked, had to be completed no matter what.

The thing that made it farcical was that the electronic booking programme we used had an inbuilt feature that prevented the overbooking of lists based on the average time any individual surgeon took to do that type of operation.

In our system, at the time of my employ, that feature was allegedly disabled so that we could deliberately overbook lists.

In order to model the running of a theatre suite and determine root causes for the stressors that were occurring, I made up a game.

It was a simple game. I called it 'Surgery Stat!'.

If the pathway from novice to expert for a clinician is a journey of learning to identify trends from their early patterns, then it is no less so for a manager.

The pathway from novice to expert is a pathway of learning, and if a manager is going to learn, they need the tools and the reflective apparatus with which to learn.

The reason clinicians get smashed repeatedly, the reason an operating theatre is a phoenix operation, worked to death each day, and rebirthing at the new dawn, is because we refuse to learn.

We refuse to learn the implications of disrespecting the limits of our time, infrastructure and human resources.

Surgery Stat! is a game that allows iconic visual identification of operating resource boundaries.

It constructs a reflective model as a learning experience and affords a way of revising what sentinel decision-making nodes went awry (or right) in review.

Conflict at the front desk occurs simply because different people with different vested interests interpret poorly delineated data from the perspective of their own cognitive bias.

It finishes up being a 'tragedy of the commons' if boundaries are not adequately defended and equity is not fairly triaged.

For the game, see www.belowtenthousand.com

Then make up your own model and see what you think.

Malicious Compliance

In a drill in a nuclear power station, operators got bored with trying to communicate with their instructors about the best way to handle a particular situation.

In the end, since no one was listening to what they were saying, the operators decided simply to test what the instructors were stipulating, despite their concerns.

When the simulation commenced, they rigorously followed the instructions they had been given by their instructors and rode the nuclear core all the way to meltdown.

In debrief, they were charged with 'maliciously following instructions'.

I've read two novels on malicious compliance, both, interestingly enough, from Eastern Europe.

The Good Soldier Švejk by Jaroslav Hašek.

And *The Life and Extraordinary Adventures of Private Ivan Chonkin* by Vladimir Voinovich.

Both are laugh out loud funny, and both involve the lowest ranking soldiers simply following their instructions to the letter of the law.

The latter allegedly so embarrassed the Soviet authorities that they refused to allow publication in Russia.

The idea of standing around watching stupid people afforded a modicum of power trying to think is enough to remind us that science is not enough.

The art of applying intelligence to any situation lies in the art of thinking.

Švejk and Chonkin should resonate with nurses familiar with the fact that simple measures innovated through the sweat and tears of immersion in the clinical interface often fall on deaf ears.

Simple measures like fatigue management, engineering barriers to overutilisation and developing an architecture which improves the flow of clumsy systems of work.

Simple measures that finish up being regarded as no more than banter and which, having failed to gain traction, mean you have no choice but to engage in what you know to be a farcical absurdity with the good grace of a smile and a numb brain, whilst those in power remain stunned by the complexity of it all, ignorant of the fact that the unfathomable complexity is underscored by very simple elements in a very simple algorithm.

To remain Authentic in such a situation is effortful. Part of you deep inside cannot help but die with the embarrassment of it all.

Dead Man's Anchor

When I look around me, at the content on Patient Safety Learning's 'The Hub', on Reddit or on LinkedIn, it seems that every nursing forum wants change.

Better still, there is a plethora of information on how to be a great nurse, how to be an inspiring, empowering leader, what to do so that the clinical interface is more effective.

It's everywhere.

So the question I ask is ...

"What is holding us back?"

In my home hospital, from which I am now retired, I will allege the ones holding us back were our administrators.

Their seemingly hostile approach to human relations, their strangling grip featuring command and control leadership were administrative paradigms most popular in the 1940s, and seemingly resurgent now.

In a desperate attempt to brutalise their workers into performance, they created a workplace environment that was little better than a gulag.

Ivan Denisovich's guard mindlessly wiping the grease off his hands onto Ivan's uniform is a stark image of mindless, needless and pointless disregard.

In a new era where patients and nurses feel empowered to insist on the presence of a safety culture in the delivery of their care, such an administration has no place.

The thing that is holding us back is an administration with too few skills to propel us into the safety culture that nurses and patients so desperately want.

A 'just' culture is all we ask.

If you can't handle that, get out of the clinic.

Soil

As a farmer, I have discovered one simple fact.

That fact is this:

That if you care for the soil, the plants will grow all by themselves.

That is, that if you take proper care to build the best substrate possible, and then insert the seed and add a little water, growth of the plant takes care of itself, all by itself.

Sustainable systems behave in the same way.

If you take care that you have created the most appropriate substrate; and if you take care to work out the macro and micro inputs needed, and account for them, then the output occurs all by itself.

If you are repeatedly dealing with crisis after crisis, then an element which should be in your systems model is missing and your calculation is flawed.

You don't need to get it right first go, but working with incremental gains will prove that sound systems optimise at the lowest energy input that still yields a sustainable output.

Note:

Trying to outperform the market does not work.

Shortcuts lead only to moonshots that crash on take-off.

To perform well in a market, it is imperative that you understand the market and all its permutations intimately.

Otherwise it is all down to luck.

The saying "It is better to be lucky than good," is fine, but we wouldn't want it to be the central tenet of healthcare, would we?

Therapeutic Window

The graphic representation of the therapeutic window should be familiar to most nurses.

It is often used to illustrate the plasma concentration of a drug, most commonly a narcotic, to demonstrate the attainment of the therapeutic window, the level at which analgesia is most effective.

Not enough drug and the patient experiences toxic levels of pain, too much and the patient experiences side effects like sedation, respiratory depression, nausea and vomiting.

The therapeutic window is achieved most commonly through incremental gains, and the most effective dose becomes apparent as the medication reaches its most therapeutic level.

Of course there are lots of other phenomena that get in the way of adequately treating pain, but as a graphic representation, the model above will do.

I have used this model to illustrate my concept of sustainability in work systems, because it seems to fit.

Clunky systems of work, overutilisation of finite resources and a lack of respect for the sustainability of the system result in pain.

Incremental gains through improving systems of work, work flow and respecting the boundaries of the resources puts you at optimal performance.

Go too far, try too hard to outperform the market and the system suffers a treacherous malaise.

Most people, given the side effects of narcotics when treating acute pain, often say they preferred the pain.

Authenticity is about reaching and maintaining that sustainable window.

Once you are there, you will be surprised at how little effort it takes for a vigilant manager to keep things there.

But don't get too comfortable.

Take your foot off the pedal and you will soon be back into that world of pain.

Microclimates

If you are exhausted, it takes exceptional poise to be able to step back and engage in your own wellbeing.

The 'Edge of Coping' is about exploring the landscape around sustainability in work performance expectations, and I am sad to say that I have spent more time thinking about that unfortunate construct.

If it is not enough to have to care for everyone else, we are told we have to care for ourselves as well.

And if, in caring for others, there is no reciprocity, as is often the case, then we are stranded in very hostile territory.

But let's let loose another thought:

What if all the expectations demanded of us were within the limits of sustainability?

What then?

What then is that any problems that still occur are for the individual to own and transcend, part of the background existential psychology that makes us who we are, not who we want to be.

If you are so in demand that you don't get time for your 'self', how on earth are you going to be able to get even close to identifying, dissecting and healing those parts of you that are getting in your own way of your own desired future identity?

The 1.5 Metre Rule

John Gibbs' 1.5 Metre Rule was famous amongst his colleagues, and it arose long, long before Covid.

The 1.5 Metre Rule was his way of protecting himself against his own sensory acuity, his own sense of vigilance in his (and once, OUR) workplace.

In John's working world, his perioperative environment, the time and effort he put into his nursing Authenticity and integrity was so eroded by the carnage extracted on his utility reward by his managers that the effective space around him regressed to 1.5 metres.

No much more than just one extended arm's reach of circumference around his person.

If you are ever in John's position, for whatever reason, you will know what he means.

John is lucky. He has an awesome family around him to offer support, but not all are so lucky.

For people with existential challenges both at work AND at home there is precious little respite.

Whatever your situation in addition to a hostile work culture: maybe an abusive relationship, caring for young children, caring for elderly parents, balancing finances or just the myriad complexities that form the living of daily life … the contraction of your world, that is your effective, rational space, warps in, shrink wraps you, as the relentless absurdity that envelops you in every direction constrains your emotional world so that your tears commingle with the shrinking baste of your own logic and the only thing you can control is your own 1.5 metres.

The Fractal Nature of Circles of Influence

Circles of influence are fractal.

A circle of influence is the radius centred around yourself that you influence in your day to day existence.

The circle thus formed represents the limit of your power.

Fractal means repeating patterns on different scales.

Nature has fractal dimensions.

As an example, if you look at a tree, you will find a repeating pattern on different scales. The trunk of the tree and the primary branches is a pattern that is repeated on a diminishing scale all the way up to the terminal twigs.

According to mathematicians, many things in nature have a two-dimensional fractal dimension of 1.2 to 1.6.

Jackson Pollack painted in fractals.

His work can be sequenced according to when it was painted in his career.

At first he painted slightly looser than nature at a fractal dimension of 1.1, but by the end of his run his work, as represented by *Blue Poles*, for example, bore a fractal dimension of 1.72, a tighter fractal dimension than nature.

Funnily enough, Pollack knew nothing about fractals.

Some would say he knew nothing about painting.

But the value of his work remains, not the least because it brought accessibility to art, the courage to find self-expression in paint, to so many.

So if Jackson Pollack's fractal dimensions were vital to the progression of art, John's fractal dimensions are no less vital to progressing the Authenticity of nursing for nurses.

It goes a bit like this:

In the beginning there is a circle of influence.

The circle of influence is the effective reach of a person.

There are three predominant sizes: the regressor, the progressor and the transgressor.

The regressor is a disempowered victim, a person who has a circle of influence that only includes themselves and the 1.5 metres. They seek respectability through mere survival.

The transgressor is a bully who is on a trajectory of overt gain. They can only get where they are going by transgressing the boundaries of others. To bully a person, a minority or a race, you must first find a reason to invalidate them. Once you have invalidated them in your own mind, to deprive them of all material and social worth is a victimless crime.

The diameter of the bully's circle of influence is a virtual Ground Zero Blast Radius. The Blast Radius is dictated by whatever megatonnage they can weaponise in their effort to construct an edifice in honour of themselves.

Ultimately they seek respectability through hostile acquisition. And despite the destruction that surrounds them, they want to be valued for the sense of self-importance they have accumulated.

The progressor, on the other hand, holds the middle ground. The progressor is on a trajectory of establishing identity through intrinsic value, Valuing the self as well as honouring the intrinsic Authenticity of others.

Progressors are custodians who seek respectability through benevolence. They create a celebration of the efforts of others, visible through the efforts of their utopian collaboration.

In the end it is possible to see these fractal dimensions all around you, whether you stand in an operating theatre or not.

Look around and tell me what you think.

Getting back to the original puzzle, a progressor culture starts to look a bit like this:

(This is what I want so that John can expand his 1.5 metres to a more comfortably sized and more empowering safe zone.)

I want his environment to celebrate John's Authenticity.

I want a culture that will celebrate who John truly is.

I want what he has to offer to see light of day in a dynamic, benevolent and progressive world where great things are possible simply because we choose NOT to shit on each other but choose to live up to the title that was once bestowed upon us: Homo sapiens, 'wise man'.

Because John, in the right environment, can not only empower himself; he can empower others to achieve well beyond belief.

And that is a legacy truly worthy of a pilgrimage!

Integration of a Safety Culture

What draws people to nursing is their search for Authenticity.

In amongst their immersive journey from novice to expert they find a pathway to stress inoculation.

They find the passion to aspire, the patience to learn the skills and techniques they need, the practice to transcribe those skills into competencies and the perseverance to further embed their skills into mastery.

Finally they have the passion to mentor others so that others may share in the joy of successfully traversing their own journey.

Infusing each of these stages are the Authentic essences of trust and technique.

And yet, dwelling like a fog within the marshes of progression is a cloud of bullying, fatigue, overwhelming production pressure and a gross ethical burden which threatens to bog the Authentic journey at every turn and turn it toward a slough of despond.

And whilst the cloud seems an absolute obstacle, it represents, in fact, an amazing opportunity.

The opportunity within production pressure is to make a strategic choice: to resource or restrain the workload.

The opportunity within the bias of bullying is to integrate a safety culture.

The opportunity in fatigue is to set boundaries around the science of human performance limitations.

The opportunity within the ethical burden is to triage systemic futility out of the duty of care.

We can't do everything for everyone.

That is the limit of our duty of care.

Rather than invalidating nurses and thus turning the brutality of performing healthcare at the clinical interface into a victimless crime, we should honour what it takes to do a good job, hence restoring Authenticity and integrity back into the frontlines of care.

The Bully Bell

We've always seemed to think of bullying as a person on person phenomena. At least, that's how we try to deal with it in healthcare organisations I have worked for.

Conflict resolution, therefore, is seen as managing two people: the deflated victim and the inflated perpetrator.

From my perspective our method is flawed and thus doomed to failure. I see bullying as being a social problem, a cultural blight, and the successful management of bullying is to understand the Bullying Bell Curve.

Any of the social sciences will teach the mathematics of the normal population distribution curve.

It is simple and easily understood.

In a bullying culture, at the centre of the curve, right in the middle, resides the queen bee. Around the queen bee are the drones who give validity to her sense of royalty. They deliver her the emotional sustenance she requires, do her bidding in order to prove loyalty and thus remain within her protective sphere of influence.

It is not a bad place to be, because you fall within the realms of control of the seemingly most powerful person in the local population.

The highest risk place to be is in the intermediate zones. You are exposed because you fall within the queen bee's hunting ground. You either desire to belong in the inner circle, or you have not yet proven yourself to be of zero worth to the bullies.

Counterintuitively, the most peaceful place to dwell is in the very outer margins. There, happily, you are either too far in exile or too strong to be considered worthy prey. You may be made fun of, but the words and the behaviours have no sting. You have become stoic. You do not react to taunts and are therefore immune.

Therefore bullying is not a one to one phenomenon any more than a symptom is the disease.

Bullying is a cluster problem within a population of remorseless sociopaths, passive observers, and confused victims.

Patterns of behaviour are not linear. They ebb and peak. The most dangerous time is when you have dealt with a conflict and washed your hands of it, thinking, "Thank god that's done."

What follows is only a temporary truce for the purposes of recuperation and rearmament, not an end of all bullying.

Worse, the bullying cohort may have learned something in the process that allows them to escalate behaviour and act with more impunity, a greater inner surety, next time.

In a domestic relationship this is known as a cycle of violence:

Expressions of endearment to drag the victim closer, followed by building resentment followed by an eruption of rage followed by expressions of endearment all over again, with each cycle getting more powerfully violent, more intrinsically corrosive, the only effective protection being to have the courage to leave.

Zero tolerance is a fine phrase, but it is of delusional worth. It makes us more ashamed, and therefore more willing to discredit the truth. The problem is not one of attaining the mystical value of zero, because we are easily fooled and we let ourselves down. Time restraints and poor competence means that reporting becomes risky, follow up fails and due process is lost to time.

Because bullying is a natural human behaviour, the brake occurs through empowering the culture of the social group, and coaching the resilience of both ends of the spectrum.

The victim is the first person to highlight the problem, usually as a cry for help.

Increasing their resilience and feelings of self-worth, helping them understand that bullying is a failure of logic that leads to conflict, and giving them realistic faith in the effectiveness of the system and the support it provides is good.

Equally, coaching the perpetrator with regards to inter-personal boundaries, decommissioning their overactive emotional radar; and managerial skill in performing the effectiveness of formal leadership structures will help at the other end.

Bullies grow because of a void in leadership. A small group decides to take on aggressive performance appraisal as their own inept right.

Such behaviour escalates to conflict, and the phenomenon will recur forever into the future because it is a quintessential part of our baboon-like nature.

Zero tolerance is a furphy.

It gives us an unrealistic aim, a reassurance that each event is the last.

Which is so not true.

Eternal vigilance and growing the emotional intelligence of both ends of the spectrum is the only solution.

The victim and the perpetrator are merely red flags, warning signs that more work needs to be done.

Instead, we want to turn the Bullying Bell Curve around.

We want the main population in the normal distribution curve to possess emotional intelligence.

We want the main population to model affirmative character traits.

We want those people to actively defend the boundaries of social decency.

And we want them to teach those who would learn, to be the best they can be.

Protecting the boundaries of decency requires emotional intelligence over bullies and zealots.

Bullies and zealots? Because anyone who expects perfection from anyone, including themselves, transgresses what is humanly possible and sets up the hell that is elitism.

Protecting the boundaries of decency? Because anybody who is a lazy enough thinker that they would erode Authenticity by demanding fatigue from overwork, or frustration of the sensibilities by enforcing overburdening and poor systems of work is a bully just as those with sociopathic egocentricities become bullies.

We want bullies and zealots to be relegated to the margins where they belong, beyond the hard deck boundaries of decency.

Emotional intelligence will lead us to the place we want to be, a culture where we can practise with Authenticity within the limits of psychomotor performance and within a system of work designed around the architecture of sustainability and do-ability, where ordinary people can work well within the limits of their growing competencies and walk away each day feeling empowered about working in a career which is the best in the world, the career that defines the pinnacle of humanity with an ethic engineered to ease the burden of suffering irrespective of wealth, race or creed.

It's not too much to ask, is it?

White Cow

A diamond sun rises over the completely dry Everlasting Swamp. It breaks through the winter mist, but the cold fingers of dawn add no warmth to the bleak landscape.

It is officially the worst drought in recorded history, and 98% of New South Wales is affected.

On the New England Tablelands, not two hours away, you can drive for miles without seeing a single live animal. There is no water. There is no grass.

The fact that people still live on their properties is testament to the fact that farming is a survival economy.

The mathematics of agriculture is a top-down calculation, not a bottom-up one.

When you buy beef or milk from a supermarket, the price set is what executives, shareholders and profiteers think the market will bear.

They work on an economy of scale and they are very sensitive to the fact that shoppers are price-sensitive.

Then, farmers sell to them at auction price through their local sale yards.

Farming is one of the few industries that buy at retail value, sell at wholesale value, and pay the freight both ways.

Prices vary based on supply and demand and vary from week to week, season to season, year to year.

The whole system is set up to be inhumane to animals.

It takes $250 to raise a single calf to weaning age. That is if it is looked after well and suckles the whole time on a cow that has adequate age, health and nutrition.

Overheads and depreciation costs are extra.

So if a farmer doesn't get much more than that cost for the animal's soul at the sale yards, neither cow nor calf is going to be looked after well.

Farmers are going to cut corners and gamble with animal health, and they are going to feel vindicated in doing so.

My old man has this internal struggle going on. It is a problem of definition. He can't work out if his farm is a hobby or a business. When cattle prices are low, it is a hobby. When cattle prices are high, it is a business. His business model is a survivalist one.

In truth, farmers' wealth depends for the most part on merely occupying the land for years on end and waiting for it to appreciate in value.

They are more land value speculators than they are custodial businesses.

In the meantime, if you want to make money out of farming, make money out of farmers. Farmers will spend what money they have at the local produce store on seed, feed, fertiliser, herbicides, machinery and fences to the point of going broke.

In a produce store, all they care is that the farmer pays their bill. It is the farmer who gambles on risk.

If you think the farmers are hard done by, consider the cows. They are merely a production unit poorly supported on lowest cost. They roam the paddocks in good years and bad, snapping off the shortest blades of grass with nothing but their teeth and tongue.

Every year they have a new calf, often having no rest between weaning last year's calf and dropping this year's, because the price at the sale yards is based on weight and the clever farmer will know that every day and every kilo counts.

With the current drought, at the end of winter the grass bears as much edible sustenance as a carpark, and yet the herd continues on.

Watching the White Cow, I wonder how she nibbles away the blades of grass she manages to tug from the earth. I try to give her extra—an extra bit of hay here, some green grass I've picked from the side of the road there, a bit of molasses to give her energy to keep grazing …

But it's not enough. Eventually this old, beautiful cow, who has put up with so much, is too weak to walk far in order to graze, and finally, too weak to stand.

As she struggles to get to her feet in order to continue on, the skin gets worn from her knees and underbelly and sores appear. It pains me to watch her.

There are no good times ahead. There is no rain predicted this spring.

With her age and the poverty of drought, there is no chance of recovery. There is only the certainty of extended suffering.

I make the decision early. She is not my cow. Technically, she belongs to the old man. I have no authority, really, but to stand and watch.

I know the old man will linger in his attempts to make her stand, bear a new calf, watch it struggle as she has no milk to feed it, and watch the suffering descend deeper and deeper in White Cow's eyes until only the sockets are staring pitifully back at me.

So I act out of my own Authenticity, early, decisively, humanely. Much to the old man's rage when he finds out what I have done.

Bang. Bang.

One shot to the middle of the forehead. The second shot to the back of the head, to the brainstem.

The first to kill. The second to make sure.

I don't wait so see her in her death throes. I leave her mates to mourn. And if you don't think cows can mourn, then you don't know cows.

Don't know cows at all.

Top Down

Nursing is a lot like farming.

The economic calculations are made from the top down.

By politicians, shareholders, executives and profiteers.

The nurses at the patient care interface don't get a look in as far as the calculations are concerned.

For a nurse, as much as it is for White Cow, the economics are survival economics. You only get what you need to survive in the gamble that you will remain productive. And should you succumb, hit hard times, with your long-suffering demise a new nurse will take your place.

Many managers know they don't have the skills to do a damn thing about it. All they can do is occupy their seat until retirement in the certainty that, being one step removed from the production line, they, at least, hold the gun.

I've seen plenty of White Cows in nursing.

I liked Inge. She always turned up with a smile on her face and a readiness to do whatever was needed. When she fell, a consequence of having her foot run over by an anaesthetist in a hurry with a patient on a theatre trolley, Inge was replaced by Sally.

I liked Sally. She always turned up with a smile on her face and a readiness to do whatever was needed. When Sally fell with a career ending back injury from pushing trolleys on a carpeted corridor with too large a friction component, her prior expressions of concern laughed off by her bosses, Sally was replaced by Leyland.

I like Leyland. He always turns up with a smile on his face and a readiness to do whatever is needed. When I see Leyland, I often wonder: Where does our duty of care to Leyland lie when we have failed our duty of care to his two predecessors?

Are we so blind to the consequences of our poor governance that we see the innocent Inges and Sallys and Leylands as dispensable, so long as there is someone else to become cannon fodder in their place?

Laws exist to prevent harm in the workplace. But they are useless if we pay no heed to them.

Ignored, they do not help us improve our governance of safety, and they certainly didn't help Inge and Sally.

Worse, people like Inge and Sally become double victims because they are forced to leave the work they love and put so much of themselves into, and are soon forgotten by people they thought of as their 'friends'.

In some places, the organisational policy seems to scream:

"We will use you up, and when we have used up the very last drop of your vitality, do us a favour: don't share with us your suffering. Just go away quietly and die."

For Inge and Sally, their will to do good was turned against them, corporatised and monetised and fed back to them as dot points on a KPI chart.

I wonder each time I see Leyland: "What preventable harm will fall to him?"

Fallen angels with broken wings find it difficult to fly out of purgatory.

Crabs

In a boat at Red Rock, Greg was collecting crabs.

I wondered why he didn't put the lid on his bucket.

"There is no need," he said. "Whenever a crab makes it to the lip of the bucket, the other crabs always pull him back in."

None of the crabs ever make it to freedom because of the critical mass of crabbiness in the bottom of the bucket

So do crabs deserve their collective fate? To be plunged alive into boiling water?

And similarly, do nurses deserve their fate of being plunged alive into burnout by a critical mass of nurses who refuse to consider any improvement to their human factors environment, any other alternative to the bucket of their present reality?

The light of Florence Nightingale's lamp beckons forth our Authenticity.

Yet we hide at the bottom of the bucket and declare that all nurses forever should share our stolid fate.

Cognitive Laboratory

Robert Frost, great American poet, is working on the stone fence between two orchards with his neighbour when he ponders what the fence is there for at all.

The things that stop us from moving forward in the operating theatre are no less perplexing than Robert Frost's wonder at the need to repair a redundant fence.

The cognitive landscape is not framed around logic, but rather the refusal to engage in logic.

In the operating theatre, our teetering rock fence is our refusal to avail ourselves of the benefits of incorporating human factors into our thought processes as well as our work.

It is as though we blindly continue on, wearing our fingers to the bone, simply to save ourselves the effort of reengineering our systems of work into something that will phenomenally improve outcomes for everybody.

Closer to home, it is like me being too busy hammering away at felling a tree to stop and sharpen my axe.

Which is why John Gibbs, Rob Tomlinson and I collaborate in the way we do to accomplish the things we do.

It might not seem like much, but in the end, the correct divisions of labour and the willingness to share in order to explore is what makes the Below Ten Thousand Way work.

I have the time to write, so I write.

I use the combined experiences of other people to inspire and infuse my words. John and Rob are still professional career nurses. They both perform in what we have come to see as the 'Cognitive Laboratory' of the workspace, the operating theatre floor.

Separated by 16,000 kilometres of continents and oceans, we still get to work together to envision a reengineered and empowered future based around how we, as nurses, do the things we do.

Of course, nothing simple is ever easy. People have minds of their own, and they aren't afraid to use them.

I remember, as occupational health and safety representative, looking one day at the way we moved patients from their theatre trolley to the operating table.

I could see the inefficient pathways and the confusion that led from people being in the wrong place during the simple act of transferring the patient.

The anaesthetic nurse stood on the trolley side, the theatre tech stood next to the anaesthetic machine, the anaesthetist stood at the drug trolley drawing up anaesthetic drugs and the scout nurse counted instruments, and no one was in charge of the move.

For a job that required a minimum of four people to be smooth and safe, two people were on the opposite sides of the movement to where they should be, and the other two were often disengaged from the process altogether.

With the patient now on the operating table, the theatre tech and the anaesthetic nurse had to walk around the theatre, keep from bumping into each other, navigate the machinery and the sterile setup, in order for the tech to move the trolley out of the room and the anaesthetic nurse to start connecting the patient to the anaesthetic machine monitoring, sort out the tubing and get ready for intubation.

Access and egress, not to mention teamwork, effort and safety, were much compromised when all that needed to happen was for the tech and the nurse to swap positions, and the anaesthetist and the scout nurse to privilege the moment.

So simple, so logical, and yet … so impossible to implement. Even when people had run out of excuses, they simply finished up in the wrong place through sheer habit.

So if Robert Frost thought he had a problem mending wall, how much worse is it when one hundred patient transfers per day, a fair percentage of them bariatric, get undertaken in a way that confounds logic, not to mention patient and staff safety?

The cognitive laboratory finishes up being challenged by something very different to what we thought it would be.

It finishes up not being a work design problem, though that is the ultimate aim. It finishes up being a person problem: how to sell human factors change to intelligent people who can't and won't change their minds.

It is a question the wonderful poet Elizabeth Barrett Browning grappled with when she posed the following question: "Can you change a person's mind against their will?"

In the end, you have to change their will against their mind, and allow their headspace to catch up.

It's not an easy thing to do.

Cognitive behavioural therapy is founded pretty much on this simple concept.

And yet, the refusal to change can be inexplicably absolute.

Clinicians have to WANT to change. If only they would stop DOING for the briefest moment so they could think, just once, about what they were doing.

This is what we have learned in our cognitive laboratory. We have the knowledge. We have the expertise. And yet our own colleagues refuse, even for a second, to stop pushing and pulling against each other (and, even more determinedly, against us) in the belief that their incomprehensible struggle is all for the greater good.

Looks like you can lead a horse to water. But you still need to feed it salt in order to make it drink.

Clinician-led culture change is yet but an interloper, a Trojan horse into our safety culture.

We have to remind ourselves that sometimes it takes 10 or 20 years to win a battle, simply because organisational politics makes intellectually arrogant people too wary of lowly clinicians bearing gifts.

Looks like we really did sell the Below Ten Thousand concept to the world in order to sell it to our own organisation.

And it looks like, in doing so, our home hospital may finally reengineer itself to make possible the change that we tried so hard for so long to realise.

'Below Ten Thousand.' Just three simple words.

Our ultimate success will be when we metamorphose our enduring legacy from the banality of one manager's emphatic outburst when she declared:

"All you have is three words … And when you leave they will die,"

to

"Let's make those three words fly!"

Why is so simple so hard?

Mission Brown

The 'other' future of nursing leadership rests with people like Rob.

Rob has essential knowledge, the aptitude to apply it, and the fortitude to keep trying.

He also has to charisma to impart his expertise to others, to plant the seed of hope and method in their hearts in the anticipation that, if nurtured, the plant will grow.

Rob's legacy will prove to be his human factors capital. Despite his brilliance, it is not an easy task. And yet, out there beyond the borders of our cognitive laboratory, there is a world clamouring for his energy, knowledge and time.

Once he has gone, his organisation will wonder at what they have lost, although they may never have allowed themselves the good grace to tap Rob's true worth.

In the meantime, I will tell him the same words (localised to time and place, of course) I told one of my colleagues when local petty politics eroded her ability to impart her passion for excellent patient care in her own workplace:

"You have more to offer than our institution can ever give you credit for."

My colleague chose to stay, to the expense of her physical and mental health.

I pray that Rob may be more heedful of my words when I invite him to reach for the stars.

Despite the risks inherent in a journey to the unknown, to stay in a place that rusts your own vibrancy is to paint over Van Gogh's *Sunflowers* with Mission Brown.

Red Flags

Shortly after my first book *The Below Ten Thousand Way* was published, my daughter sent me a message: "Dad! You've GOT to listen to this!" She included a link to a podcast on 'Dr Death'.

The cringe factor was high. How did such a person remain in his profession, actively harming people, for so long without being challenged?

For me there was an easy answer. We are not trained in Red Flags.

In subsequent conversations over many hours, Hani and I have developed the Red Flags idea based on lived experiences and our shared strategy to deal with them over the course of both our professions.

The ability to adopt Red Flags is critical in the journey towards Authenticity. To fail to attend to Red Flags, your own and others, is to fail in Authenticity.

A Red Flag is an early warning sign, usually of a low level danger that warrants observation.

Watchful observation once behaviour makes visible a single proverbial Red Flag may reveal yet more, formerly unidentified, Red Flags.

This cluster may uncover a pattern of behaviour, which may be a symptom of a more serious underlying phenomenon, which would otherwise continue unabated should it not be detected, acknowledged and corrected.

Like 'Dr Death'.

Red Flag behaviour is a poor response to a reasonable challenge.

A Red Flag behaviour's intent is to create emotive uncertainty in the other person, either by attempting to demoralise, dominate or create overt fear.

In dealing with these situations, we usually concentrate on one Red Flag, the precipitating event.

This leaves us vulnerable to poor outcomes and repeated, often escalated behaviour by the perpetrator as time goes on.

It leaves our team susceptible to a cycle of violence which goes around in circles with the very people we try to protect being much worse off in the long run.

Counterintuitively, the perpetrator of the Red Flag behaviour sees your ineffective conflict resolution process, not as an improvement process or correctional process, but as a learning opportunity to improve the success of future attempts at manipulation in order to get their own way.

It is not a very happy picture.

There is no end to the behaviour. The end of one cycle is just the beginning of another. It is exactly the same as the cycle of domestic violence.

Roses and chocolate, followed by a build-up period, then the explosion. A resolution process of "I'm sorry, I don't know what came over me, it won't happen again, and besides, it was your fault anyway ..." then a sort of eggshell truce, before the planting of the first landmine in another field of landmines.

Sometimes our biggest failure is that we don't sack these people.

Instead, we let them leave of their own accord, and offer them a lovely, perjured reference on their way out the door.

So How do Red Flags Help?

Red Flags allow you to see an entire pattern of behaviour. They place on your desk a map of interpersonal reactions. When dealing with just one event and one behaviour, you are trivialising the behavioural roadmap.

When all behaviours are visible and on the table, the ability to dismiss the event as a one off is reinforced, especially if there are no other Red Flags, and if a root cause analysis leads to significant other factors being identified as major initiators of the event.

Even then, Red Flags become an integral part of moving forward.

In the event of interpersonal conflict, two Red Flags are immediately raised, one on behalf of the perpetrator and one on behalf of the victim.

The opportunity here is to improve the behavioural responses of the perpetrator, but also to increase the resilience of the victim.

It becomes a win-win, as both players, should they engage in the challenges laid out for them, develop skills which add value to the composite team.

Should a party choose not to engage in behavioural competencies, you may very well wonder at the viability of the relationship:

"What future is there in their continued tenure on my team?"

Because no matter how technically advanced their technical skill is, if their job is to work with other people and they lack the ability to do this, then their presence will only be destructive and cause you migraine after migraine.

Best let their genius be manifested somewhere else. Collateral damage only serves to reduce your team to rubble. And if you don't think that's a problem, you should.

Should you choose to sacrifice your team to preserve a bully, I would wonder at your own managerial competence and Authenticity, because it's not as though there is not plenty of information out there on Authentic leadership.

After a career in clinical nursing, once you take a managerial position, it seems your own professional development is up to you, and unless you chase down the skills you need, which are entirely different to the clinical skills you once thrived on, how can you be Authentic in your newly acquired role?

The Authenticity of Standards

At my last count, a few years ago now, the ACORN (Australian College of Operating Room Nurses) Standards had 58 standards and guidance statements that form a framework for safety and quality in the operating rooms.

And yet, in many places, most of them are ignored.

We may pay attention to the surgical count but dismiss staffing levels.

We may pay attention to sterile processing but dismiss wellbeing.

We may pay attention to retained items but dismiss fatigue.

And yet, despite the standards being the scaffolding that supports the very work we do, few nurses are intimately acquainted with its contents.

What hope have we got when competence is assumed despite a lack of knowledge of the standards?

An Authentic nurse would know the standards, not as a desired aspiration, but as a bottom line in need of staunch defence.

I had a young student once who had facial piercings. She was made to feel stupid by an educator on account of the infectious risks the student's piercings presented her patients.

The student was quite upset when she approached me and asked me to be her mentor for the day, and it didn't take long for me to become upset as well.

I took the student for a walk down the theatre corridor and looked into theatres where operations were being performed with open doors, where people were entering and exiting rooms in haste and where the noise and bustle created a vortex of microorganism-aerosolling activity.

At the end of the corridor we stopped in a sunlit patch by a window overlooking the bay and paused for a minute.

I'm not sure that I reassured the nurse, but my explanation went something like this:

"How dare they pick on you when you provide a low risk of harm with your personal life choice, when, every day in every way, every nurse in every theatre performs out of synch with good practice, with a subtle break in the sterile field here, picking up a dropped item off the floor there, wearing the same theatre hat, unwashed, for months if not years on end, little things that make certain that a million patients are harmed in a million small ways and which make the act of merely entering a hospital an act of bravery and misplaced trust on the patient's behalf?"

My student for the day was exceptional. Her aptitude, her attention to detail, her ability to engage with the patient were brilliant, and in fact, if she learned anything off me, it was reciprocated by me learning things off her.

For example, she was fastidious about swabbing the injection hub on a drip with an alcohol wipe, then waiting 15 seconds before injecting IV medications, something I found difficult to incorporate into my habitual practice.

Observing her embedding it so easily into her system of work made me stop and think:

"If she can do it, why can't I?"

So few anaesthetists and so few old school nurses are successful at attending to so simple an act.

This simple observation turned that statistic around.

This student, who two hours ago was being torn apart for her perceived lack of professionalism, a perceived lack of consideration of patient wellbeing, has now saved more lives through that simple re-education than the educator will ever have managed because of her habit of reinforcing poor standards merely for the fact that they were entrenched.

I think I was the first person to say to this nurse: "Do your work as you are taught. Show me the correct way, because my habits are 20 years out of date whereas yours are fresh out of school."

This nurse was a lifesaver.

She was, indeed, Authentic to her profession.

The Plimsoll Line

Most people are familiar with the Plimsoll Line. It is the line painted on the side of ships to prevent them from being overloaded.

Before the Plimsoll Line came into being, ships sank with monotonous regularity. The Plimsoll Line was made compulsory on all British ships in 1876, thereby regulating payloads to within safe margins of the freeboard in order to prevent sinking.

In operating theatres, a similar problem exists. Overwhelming workload increases risk of error.

At present we have no Plimsoll Line to tell us when enough is enough. We plough on through the day regardless, sailing with the sails set for maximum speed into the storm clouds ahead.

We appear to have no benchmarks which indicate for us the relative safety of the ship we are sailing.

Or do we?

The benchmark for a safely supported clinical operating theatre seems to exist within the Standards for operating theatre practice.

The Standards, rigorously researched and peer reviewed, set out the safe minimum standards for operating room practice including staffing levels and skill mix.

They form the Plimsoll Line for a safely supported workplace.

Should staff levels and systems of work allow for better than the minimum specified due to local variances, then the system can be considered to be well supported and their ability to meet predictably predictable contingencies robust.

Should staff levels and systems of work be insufficient to meet the standards, then the system can be considered to be unsupported and the potential for meeting predictably predictable contingencies weak.

The risk is obvious.

Once upon a time, not so long ago, overvalued, over-insured and overaged ships were lost at sea with reckless abandon, sent deliberately to their demise for the purposes of profiteering.

With death from preventable medical error the third highest cause of death simply because, I would argue, hospitals are set adrift overburdened with workload and with too few staff and planning contingencies to allow for fatigue and the predictably predictable emergent workload, are we any better?

Bring in the Plimsoll Line for healthcare. Lives are being needlessly lost whilst our planning algorithms are all at sea.

Self-care

Self-care is a search for a benevolent space within a degraded system of work.

As a concept it is a longing for the supportive behaviours of our utopian baboon colony.

Self-care is the provision for an internal tranquil resort within, in an external maelstrom of activity and demands.

Sometimes there is not enough coffee in the world sufficient to wind you up. There is not enough alcohol to wind you back down.

There is a You in there somewhere, but it is on the dark side of your moon.

People have all different ways of coping, the most common being denial.

But the only cure for fatigue is rest, and when fatigue is so advanced that the body and brain begin to usurp your very willpower, even a micro-nap can save a life: yours!

So how do we build that sanctuary in our brains, that nest upon which our attentive self can snuggle down and safely rest?

Resilience is a good word, but it takes a lot of effort and dumps all the responsibility back on the person, which makes you a double victim.

Boundaries are better.

Boundaries with graded escalation including penalties for encroachment. The endpoint is knowing when to say "No!"

As Harry, my son, tells me during one of our philosophical discourses over a midnight snack: "No" can be a sentence as well as a word. There is no requirement to rationalise your "No."

So with fatigue, it is a dangerous judgement that you make if you want to start second guessing your psychomotor competence.

The simple answer is that evidence exists which fully supports your right to say "*No!*"

Enough is enough.

And whilst the 'heroic' model of care demands you give everything you have and more, and seeks to reassure you that you can do it, the rational model of care should insist that a marathon is not a sprint, nor even a series of sprints.

It is a preservation of energy in order to allow your willpower and your muscles to get you, unharmed, to the finish line.

Should you be asked to do more in order to prop up a degraded system? No.

You shouldn't even be asked, because it is categorically too dangerous a territory. It is valuing the ruin too highly And valuing yourself too lowly. Contingency plans are the mathematics of failure.

Whilst contingency planning is vital, it is better to have resilient systems of work in place so that contingencies stay where they need to be: as contingencies, not rescuers of poor systems of work and out-of-date work design.

Human factors. That's where the resilience needs to lie. Not in you as a worker.

We can't expect perfection of people. That's asking too much. But we *can* design systems of work that permits you to perform well whilst still being ordinary.

That way, we adequately value your Authenticity, your right to be a *person* as well as your right to be a *professional*.

And knowing you, you always desire to be the best that you can be.

But with everything under control, nobody needs a hero.

Bricks and Mortarboards

When you enter a hospital, be it as a patient or a member of staff, an interesting thing happens. The glass doors close behind you and you are irretrievably in a different existential space. Outside, beyond that threshold is the material world. But inside you are a new Jonah having been swallowed by a mammoth whale.

I'm interested in exploring that existential space in the interests of quantifying the healing environment.

I guess my theory is that healing doesn't start in the ward or the operating theatre or the ICU. It starts in the corridor.

There is so much happening in that simple shared space. It is where a hospital really declares itself.

The patient information plastered on the walls challenges patients to believe they are underqualified. The labyrinth reminds them that they are novice travellers in a stark strange world.

Conversations overheard, sights and sounds and smells all contribute to the feeling that they are trespassing in a world beyond their control and understanding. What does being in a hospital corridor speak of to you?

I'm going out on a limb here. I'm going to say that as hospital employees, we are taught jobs. We are not taught how to be custodians of a shared space that aspires to heal.

The way we converse in a lift, the way we smile, or not, at strangers and the way we stop, or not, when we sense that someone is lost, all counts towards the metrics of an organisational culture.

Healing is a subconscious process as well as a physiological one. Engagement starts with the sum total of all these inputs, and whether that sum total is positive or negative.

I'm happy to be wrong about this, but I'm equally happy to be right.

Share your experiences and thoughts and let's see how valuable the lived experience is in comparison to just the bricks of the building and mortarboards of our professions.

Tragedy of the Commons

The idea of the commons heralds from English village life, where if you had a sheep, you could graze it on common village ground.

Everybody in the village had equal right to the common ground, and the supposition was that if everyone behaved fairly and within the boundaries of decency, the common would provide for the needs of all.

Unfortunately, that's a big ask of human nature, and so the tragedy of the commons became a term to illustrate overutilisation of a shared public domain.

Where utopians fail in the consideration of such explicit benevolent functions is to assume that everybody is just like them.

It is an error made by Plato in his 375 BC discourse, *The Republic*, and an error refurbished by Saint Sir Thomas More in *Utopia*, published in 1516. It is also an error made by me now.

In the operating theatre, the tragedy of the commons occurs because operating theatre time, and with it, infrastructure, equipment and human resources, is a finite and increasingly precious resource.

It is an open access resource for both surgeons and patients.

Under pressure of demand from a populace demanding treatment for their ails and from every surgeon demanding the right to capitalise upon their skills and trade, rivalry occurs.

The rivalry is made more intense by the failure of infrastructure development to keep up with escalating community population growth, just as spectacularly as it fails to keep pace with the demand caused by a proliferation of emergent and elective surgical innovations.

Under intense pressure from both political and local forces, governance of the sustainable limits of this healthcare resource wilts as waiting lists become enduringly unfathomable.

In attempting to do everything for everyone, the limits of the resource become exceeded and the resource suffers to the point of degradation.

If you work in an operating theatre you will know what I mean.

The surgical environment degrades to the point beyond which it is safe, and yet we soldier on.

Safety Culture becomes overburdened, and symptoms like bullying, blaming, the taking of systemic short cuts and the overt oppression of those who would complain appear and cement themselves as the new default and expressly tangible UnSafety Culture.

Equipment becomes old, poorly maintained and prone to breakdown.

Mandatory Overtime, on-call before days off, crap rosters, and demands upon your time that exceed the boundaries of endurance, become the norm as the expectation arises that you belong to the company, not that your presence at work is just one choice you make as part of the sum total of choices in the effort to build a well-crafted, well-balanced and aspirational life.

In short, you become overburdened, dissatisfied and relentlessly fatigued simply because your managers failed to see the operating list each day as the manufactured workload it is.

You see, we get so used to allowing the idea of the emergency case, which can happen at any time, to so dominate our thinking that we assume that EVERY case is an emergency and behave accordingly.

Emergent semi-elective surgeries occupy on average 30% of our operating theatre workload, and often are performed after hours.

In 'Surgery Stat!', the game, despite there being 80 hours of elective surgical time throughout the day, we continually worked our elective lists past session times, thus consigning the more critical emergency surgery cases to late evening and well into the night.

So we couldn't do our elective surgery lists in the 80 hours allotted to them, and insisted in stealing time from the ten hours of evening surgical time allocated to time critical cases that emerged through the day.

The silly thing is that an elective operating list is a *manufactured* workload. It is pre-booked and scheduled a month in advance. And yet, despite all the metrics available, we couldn't hit our productivity targets with any degree of proficiency.

So much for surgical precision.

In fact, our governance team made it certain that we would fail every day to meet our elective surgery workload by deliberately ignoring decision-making algorithms that would alert them to the fact that theatre lists were being overbooked.

A trained eye can look at a theatre list, look at the surgeon and anaesthetist and the types of operations scheduled for the day and predict which lists would run over with a certainty much more accurate than the Bureau of Meteorology.

And yet, day after day, the pattern would be repeated.

Other forces were in play.

Department of Health penalties applied for surgeries not undertaken within certain timeframes and so, in our cleverness, workarounds were invented to hide non-compliance.

Add that cultural underbelly to the angst that cancellation caused to patients, and the anger of surgeons to the fact that their case had been cancelled, and it took a brave person to cancel an operation because we were out of time, *and* a brave person to face the fury of the executive class the next day to 'please explain'!

Surgeons booking cases act as lone agents seeking to access the commons of the operating theatre, and, acting in their own self-interests, succumb to the confirmation bias that privileges their own decision-making matrix.

Add to that their position of power and you have at the front desk of theatre a dynamite setting for stress, an explosive time critical decision-making forum, and a powder keg of vested interests primed to erupt at the earliest spark.

Every manipulation is allowable, and if cajoling and pleading doesn't work, a tantrum just might.

The nurse is the meat in the sandwich.

The extra pay isn't worth the paracetamol you need for your headache.

Max

Max* was a nurse.

He was an exceptionally good one, and he was passionate about supporting his teams (that is, both his operating theatre nursing team and his beloved AFL team) and maintaining high standards of practice.

Theatre 8 was a special theatre. It was the newest, best theatre in his complex at the time, and it was the theatre that funnily enough was always free when the accreditors came to visit.

Dr Two*, the deputy director of surgical services, would march the accreditors straight down the corridor, past Theatre 1, past Theatre 2, definitely past Theatre 3, past Theatres 4, 5 and 6, and straight into the only theatre which had been 'fixed' to meet infection control standards, so that they could have a good look around at their leisure.

It happened year after year.

One day, the hospital's director of infection control, Dr Four*, appeared in theatres to look at Theatre 8 for himself, to make sure its recent renovation passed inspection.

Nurse Max asked Dr Four to look at Theatre 3, the orthopaedic and emergency theatre.

At first Dr Four resisted, but eventually he had little choice because Max got him in a proverbial headlock and dragged him into the room.

Within five minutes, the theatre was decommissioned until major renovations were completed.

What Dr Four saw horrified him.

The theatre walls had holes in them that you could feel breeze flowing through. Wall surfaces were peeling off. Electrical outlets were held in place by surgical tape. The list goes on.

If you want a list of breaches of the Standards that existed, ask Mr Deedee*.

Mr Deedee was a politician, the Shadow Minister for Health at the time.

Max had sent Mr Deedee, following a chance meeting, a CD-ROM with an album full of pictures showing each breakdown in detail.

Of course, nothing eventuated. No one was interested and Max just got a name for himself as a troublemaker. A 'Rogue of Safety', so to speak.

Management finally found a reason to march Max out of the organisation. The reason was his increasingly frustrated behaviour and his inability, finally, to hold his peace.

Despite his popularity and his unrelenting pursuit of operating theatre standards, every other clinical nurse in the theatre complex watched him go without raising an eyebrow.

Nevertheless, the theatre got fixed. Who ever thought caring was easy? Authenticity sometimes comes at a price.

(*Names have been changed to protect the innocent.)

Faster, Faster
Too Busy to Care

Compassion is too rich for bottom-dollar quote healthcare.

My mum had her cataract operated on. Everything went swimmingly until just before discharge, when the surgeon had one last look in her eye.

He found a bit of cataract had been left behind.

"That happens in a small percentage of cases," he told her. A small percentage of cases?

In 30 years of surgery, that 'small percentage of cases' in my experience has, until now, equalled zero.

So what happened?

On the phone to my sister, I speculated: "Was the surgeon in too big a rush? Was he distracted? Was he fatigued from trying to schedule too many cases in a day?"

"It is funny you say that," replied my sister, "because when we chatted with the admission nurse, she said it was their busiest day ever."

Whatever it was, the interesting thing was that the surgeon passed it off as normal. "Aren't you special?" was the insinuation, and it was the insinuation my sister and father brought back with them from the hospital with a laugh to me, at home, looking after the family farm.

Mum had been rushed back in to theatre for a second operation to correct the errors of the first, with more chance of infection and a higher risk of complications, and all this on her only *good* eye, since the sight in her other eye was blotted out by macular degeneration.

Not really a laughing matter in the whole scheme of things, at least to me.

It's not such a rarity in healthcare, erasing an opportunity to learn from errors.

Errors are glossed over with certain-speak, aimed to scuttle the recognition of error.

In the end, we believe our own press, because we consider ourselves smart, certainly smart enough to outsmart an egregious production pressure and its inherent risk.

When an astronaut was questioned about the bravery required to venture into space, he asked the reporter how *he* would feel sitting his anus on a megaton of explosive put together at lowest quote. It is an interesting response, because when we enter a hospital, we envisage healing, not harm, just as an astronaut envisages stepping on the moon, not blowing up on take-off.

But faster faster is not a response to healing. It is a response to fiscal margins. The decision makers are not in harm's way.

In response to harm, we do everything possible except the very thing we need to do that would make us empirically much safer—slow down.

We buy flashy equipment, research new drugs, develop new operative techniques.

But patients, in the scheme of things, remain unimpressed by this if they are the ones that get harmed.

They just want us to do a good job, first time every time.

The system as it stands is the one roadblock to that outcome.

In a hurry, under time pressure, we leave behind part of a cataract, and laugh it off as an exception to the rule, despite all evidence to the contrary.

In the end, no matter how glossy the hospital brochure, it means nothing as an indicator of good surgical outcomes.

Even less if you no longer have the sight to see it with.

"I will stuff their mouths with gold"

Aneurin Bevan was a Welsh Labour Party politician who was the Minister for Health in the UK from 1945 to 1951. The son of a coalminer, Bevan was a lifelong champion of social justice, the rights of working people and democratic socialism. (Wikipedia)

The birth of the NHS was his genius, and to overcome criticism for his national health service by senior medical consultants, in his own words, he stuffed their mouths with gold.

It could be said, all these years on, that doctors still expect that their mouths be stuffed with gold, and from this esteemed right derives power, privilege and elitism.

The hierarchal culture in healthcare reflects this cultural reality.

Despite our protestations that we work in healthcare because it is our calling to help others, the best measure of truth comes from a virtual experiment.

In our cardiac theatre, the theatre staff all contributed to a lottery fund. It was often joked that if the team won the lottery, the next day there would not be a cardiac surgery theatre nurse left in town.

The very expression of that sentiment cuts away all the delusional bullshit. Do I nurse because it is inbuilt into my personal ethics? Or do I nurse because that is what I trained in and it helps to pay my bills?

If the former is true, then I will turn up to work the day after winning the lottery and stay at work until my timely retirement because it is my will.

If the latter is true, then as part of the fear that is the captured demographic of the mortgage belt, I will accept any conditions, no matter how destructive they may be to my physique and psyche, so long as I get my thirty dollars an hour.

In fact, I shall be fearful of jeopardising my position in any way, and will therefore turn a blind eye to any threat to my ongoing employment, no matter how personal it seems.

Giving lower order team members a voice, therefore, means that you have to make them feel safe and supported, as well as giving them every opportunity to practise graded escalation of engagement in a safety culture free from hierarchical constraints.

'Below Ten Thousand' is such a thing, because it gives clinicians every chance to build their advocating cognition and their vocal strength.

Every time its use is met with behavioural compliance the safety culture grows stronger because once your voice is empowered in lower-order advocacy, it becomes more certain that the group will engage equally assertively in response to higher order safety threats.

This is why Rob Tomlinson is the most important person in the NHS this millennium.

Because bravery is not a single event.

Bravery is a pattern of behaviour, and Rob is coaching clinicians, nurses just like him, in safe systems of work that empower just such a pattern of behaviour.

Enabling Advocacy

In the consideration of any journey, there is no place to start like home.

So it is only in my former department, with my former bosses, that I can consider setting out on the journey towards enabling advocacy.

So, given where I have been and what I have seen, one question forms in my mind: "Was it an alleged dereliction of authentic duty, or just poor management skills?"

In other words, to be fair, even my bosses may have just been victims of a system, and in the worst of all conundrums, may merely, themselves, have been victims of the poor succession planning typical of nursing in some places.

The benchmarks of key performance drivers are not hard to imagine.

There seem to be three main jurisdictions of a nurse manager in the operating theatre.

These fit into the categories of legislated drivers, organisational drivers, and operational drivers.

At the top end are the legislated baselines which comprise the minimum standards a manager must uphold.

Each document contains the behavioural boundaries with which a manager must comply and which they must defend, whether they agree with them or not:

First there is the Workplace Safety Act, which describes minimum levels for occupational health and safety.

Then there is the Equal Opportunity and Human Rights Act, which seeks to circumvent discrimination in the workplace.

In there also sits the Australian Commission on Safety and Quality in Healthcare which sets the Patient Charter of Rights and the National Safety and Quality Health Service Standards.

Then there is the Nursing and Midwifery Board of Australia regulations, which define the minimum standards for professional registration.

What follows next is the Industrial Agreement, which is renegotiated, in most cases, between the nurses' union and the employer representative every few years.

And finally, there are the professional standards, for example, the ACORN Standards, which form a peer reviewed best practice framework to which organisations should, but not must, subscribe.

All of this, as comprehensive and as detailed as the collective documents are, form the minimum standards managers must uphold.

In order to uphold them, one must first know them, second be motivated to aspire to them and finally, be willing to advocate on behalf of them.

To fail to do so is a failure to meet minimum standards with respect to managerial performance, which is where virtue ethics in a manager start to show.

So if you have a headache just thinking about that now, we are only getting started.

Organisational performance drivers:

- Job descriptions;
- Organisational values;
- Codes of Conduct;
- Professional scopes of practice;
- Conflict management procedures;
- Organisational procedures and policies;
- Etc.

So for each organisational objective, the greatest value in each is the behavioural expression of these objectives.

In other words, if the objectives are not upheld at every level, and not openly and fairly defended at each transgression, then they are just words on a page, or to be more specific, broken promises on a page.

Likewise, if they only apply to some and not to others, then how can there be a 'just' culture and trust in an organisation?

As a manager, it is not enough to know these objectives in detail. You must be prepared to perform them as well. Which is where values of rigour in a manager start to show.

Just in case you are feeling a little overwhelmed, don't worry. At least now we are on the homeward stretch.

Because we are now down to operational performance drivers.

For your department, as a manager you have a vision.

You also have jurisdiction over policies and procedures.

You have people management skills because management is, for the most part, about people.

You have team management skills, because it is the manager's job to form those people into teams.

You have resource management skills, because your team needs resources to do their job.

So the day to day management of workload, and the safety and quality of that work, falls explicitly on your shoulders.

The resilience, or the antifragility of your team depends upon your skills.

The day to day optimisation of a safe workload and the ability of your team to achieve the desired outcome with high reliability and due diligence relies upon your skills.

The consolidation of the team over time and the achievement of robust quality through talent identification and succession management relies upon your skills.

In the first place, anything that advances you is good. It is called incremental gain.

Then, you play the percentage game, setting a foundation of good practice and discipline upon which to build, making sure that protective policies become protective habits at all times and on all occasions for all people on your staff.

Then the behavioural and clinical rigour with which your team performs becomes a measure of your skill as a manager.

As does your ability to recruit people who are a good fit for your team over time.

Authenticity in your role? It is that simple.

Having a world class team under your management is within arms' reach. But you can't get there unless you have faith in your own vision.

If you don't have faith, and you don't have a clear vision, then you are like a leaf blowing on the wind, and the void in leadership will leave all these things up to the bullies, above, around and below you, to do as they will.

If you lack the faith to advocate on behalf of the legislation. If you lack the faith to advocate on behalf of your organisation's standards. And if you lack the faith to advocate on behalf of your peoples' rights, then sadly you are letting down the very Authenticity of your calling.

It is hard yards, the nurse's calling to ease and prevent suffering. As a manager, such a thing applies first and foremost to your staff. The flow on effect is that it will then be bestowed upon your patients.

But without the required knowledge and advocacy skills, it might as well be the sword in the stone, and it is best that you leave it alone.

Learning with Purpose

I asked my son Harry about team construction once.

We were on a drive to the tip with some rubbish, and so we had the time to talk.

Harry is famed for his Pokémon teams, and I wanted to know more about his strategy because I had hit a roadblock whilst trying to fathom skill mix, the concept of high-performance teams, and our lackadaisical attitudes towards students and novices in the operating theatre.

Haz came out with something quite profound and different to what I expected his response to be.

He constructed his team, not on sheer seniority or power, but on potential.

So he was happy to take a team with basic functional compatibilities and a portfolio of different capabilities, carefully analysed, and then he would work his team to build the capacity of his team members with latent talent into a unit of startling efficiency.

If Haz, at age 16, can give me such a profound answer, where does that leave us adults in the operating theatre?

Sadly, we would be no good at Pokémon.

READD

Students come, Students go, but the one reality in life is that there will always be another student. Some are interested, some are not so interested, and when you see a novice who is overawed and maybe a little bit frightened by the whole experience it can be hard to tell the difference.

Recovery is a hard place to be. It can seem so narrowly focussed and so immediate and so paced and so nuanced that it can be hard for them to get their heads around it all, let alone see how it fits into the broad spectrum of their overall learning experience.

Theatre is not for everyone. As a place to work, it can come off as directive, definitive, controlling, confronting. People in theatres have been trained, or at least conditioned, to communicate in a particular style:

To ask for things in a clear and concise manner, that gets them what they want when they want it and for those who don't understand that it's often ... not personal, it can be misinterpreted as being 'rude'. So, if they never want to come back, is the whole experience a waste of time?

I spend about 50% of my time in Recovery. Over time, being a clinician, I saw a number of students grasping with these very concepts, and I wondered: How do we make sense of it all for them from a uniquely 'PACU' perspective? I mean, we know what we do, and we know how and why we do what we do, and my colleagues make it look so easy.

But for someone new, the biggest problem can be that they don't know what they don't know. They can also find it difficult to work out what is important and what is not, and they may find it difficult to express that incomprehensibility in words.

One day I saw a student sitting by herself with a textbook open on page one of chapter one, looking, or rather staring and trying not to look panicked. And at the same time, not taking anything in.

She was using the most logical and rational approach in the book: Knowledge is in a textbook. When you find yourself in a strange situation, read a textbook.

For me, Chaos is a calling card. I use it to shake solutions out of problems. If you can't find the answer from within a complex rationality, it is no trouble to explore the seemingly random fractal dimensions in search of elegant simplicity.

I don't know why I trusted knowledge to chance. It's not even as though I have had that good a relationship with chance.

Let me give you an example: When I was ten ... We had the local department of agriculture release dung beetles at our farm. And I was VERY excited because dung beetles come in two types: I was hoping we would get the type that roll the manure into little balls and then roll it away to their burrows. But no. We got the sort that just buries it! Where's the fun in that?

So the dung beetles grew and grew in numbers until there were so many that the dung was buried before it even had the chance to hit the ground

And beetles would fly around the kitchen light at night ... We had visitors over for dinner one night, and as my mother was dishing up the dessert, one hit the lightbulb and dropped straight into one of the bowls of ice cream. Without even looking she scooped it out and flicked it into the corner on the room. No one saw but me ... but because I was right there and I had seen it buzzing around the light, and with prior knowledge, I'd guessed ... there was a chance ... of what was about to come.

What I didn't foresee was that she would pick up the bowl ... and hand it to me.

So somewhere in there is chance ... and knowledge, and eventually, the realisation that sometimes opportunity exists within.

I mean to say ... it was the biggest bowl of ice cream!

There has been a far longer history than that of combining chance with knowledge.

For centuries in China, the *I Ching* or *Book of Changes*, has used the toss of three coins six times to guide the application of wisdom relating to '64 known states of change'.

And so it is that I came up with the idea of the READD, of using chance and knowledge together to engage our students with strategic 'packets' of wisdom in a novel and hopefully interesting way.

In order to make it useful, on behalf of our students, I collaborated with my friend and colleague, John Gibbs, to work out:

- "What is it about Recovery that offers a unique experience?"
- "What about us offers useful skills and knowledge irrespective of where students find themselves in future?"

We wanted to know what things you get especially in Recovery. What skills we get to practise over and over, that students get less exposure to anywhere else that are transportable to the anywhere, anyhow, anytime.

What we wanted ... was the answer to this question: "What is 'Recovery' distilled down to just a few ideas?"

Given the extraordinary variance in patients, and the experiential limitations inherent within that unpredictability, the question we also had to solve was: "How can we grow a useful spectrum of knowledge for our students in a short timespan and in a meaningful way?"

So. Four suits with 13 cards.

That offered us an opportunity, and a challenge:

To develop an hierarchal stratification of elements within each conceptualised classification, so that we could layer the knowledge we expected to be able to teach and still retain enough fluidity to be able to move up or down a knowledge and skill ladder at will.

Equally importantly, we asked: "How do we prevent overload?"

John and I are happy to talk all day, but sometimes it is important to know when to stop.

Would logic suppose that ... when their nose starts running ... their brain is full? I don't know. I'm not a craniofacial expert.

However, the stratified approach means that we can pace a discussion: We can discuss a topic at will, then wait and watch for it to occur and so reinforce the principles or the skill we have been focussing on, so it can be a running topic of conversation over the course of the day, or for as long as it takes.

So three categories comprise much of the clinical and technical stuff we encounter. Cardiovascular, Respiratory, Pain: Hearts, Clubs and Diamonds.

Hearts:

It's pretty easy to see the stratification in Cardiovascular. Whether you agree with them is a different matter.

You can play Aces high or low, and so we put there the simplest and yet most profound Cardiovascular monitor we have, pulse oximetry.

It tells you when things are going right, and if you look at it in a particular way, it tells you when things are going wrong.

The information reflects a whole lot of things, obvious and subtle.

Then we stepped up to monitoring, physiology, drugs and finally arrest protocols, giving us plenty of scope to embellish or simplify any of these topics to fit the level of knowledge and experience of the student.

Once a card is picked, we start out on that topic. But as enthusiasm builds, we usually wander up and down the suit to wherever our conversation takes us.

We're happy with that. It's a knowledge exploration game, after all, not a textbook.

And we would hope not to fill them with discrete bundles of knowledge to show them how clever we are, but to inspire them to seek out clarification of, or expand upon, what we have talked about when the time ... suits them.

I mean: no one in their right mind would trust ME without checking the facts out first (not even my kids do!).

In other words, we hope to drive them back to the textbook, or even to Wikileaks, but with a clear aim, a clear purpose, and with opened eyes.

Clubs:

Looks like an alveolus, right? So, Respiratory.

Respiratory is the fun one.

It gives them something to get their hands dirty on. This is John's specialty. It's mostly anatomy and physiology, and how that translates into practice.

So it's:

- Is it easier to breathe through one straw or ten straws?
- How long can a snorkel be?
- Jaw thrust: is it torture or treatment?
- How much air should you squeeze from that two-litre bag?

- Is Lazarus Syndrome … resolved breath stacking, or is it a miracle?

And all that sort of stuff.

In the end it's fun, they learn stuff, and the whole team finishes up getting to be involved because you never know when (or who with), the next obstructed airway will occur.

Diamonds:

It looks like the tip of a scalpel, so we made this one pain.

The visual requires a leap of faith, but it's OK! Desperate situations demand desperate measures.

So if I want to talk about pain, why would I start at oximetry? I guess it is a desperate attempt by me to stick to a theme, but the unusuality of it makes it a proverbial wildcard, and that alone creates cognitive value. So long as you learn to question, THEN, you can question anything.

Aces high and Aces low. Pulse oximetry is a low-level indicator which tells me, quite subtly in the absence of any other signs, when my narcotics have hit. It's a high-level indicator of when I've gone too far.

Of course, there's more to talk about than is represented here, but what we have developed is a springboard, an introduction to the nuances of pain, it's phenomenology and its treatment as it relates to patients in Recovery.

Now I know what you are thinking. And I thought it, too: There's something not right, there's something not right, there's something not right.

I looked and I looked, and then I thought: (snap) I don't tell them where they can download their own copy of the READD.

So I put our web address on it.

www.belowtenthousand.com

And follow the links to the Recovery Education and Discussion Deck (READD)

And for a while, that satisfied me. And then, at last, I saw it. Pulse oximetry? What was I thinking?

Rule Number 1, The Universal Rule:

"Look at the patient! Look at the patient! Look at the patient!"

So how can I get myself out of such a rookie error? Truth is ... I can't. I just have to add it in now, and pretend that it was there all along.

So. That's three suits. But a deck of cards has FOUR suits, right? We ascertain that we all 'do' the clinical, the technical stuff, well.

In fact, it's all we do until a problem gets out of hand. Then we stand around, point fingers and scratch our heads.

But ... I have come to believe that technical skills should only be 3/4 of the sum total of all our knowledge.

Which brings us to Spades.

Spades:

Thirteen different ways of shovelling your way out of the shit. Survival skills for nurses.

What you can learn that will keep you, most times, out of most trouble.

We don't drill too deep, because this is an 'eye opening' process.

It's enough for us that we have introduced our students to the thought process.

Because it takes years to expose yourself to ... and assimilate this sort of information ...

So, for example, think:

7 of Spades:

What constitutes 'adequate performance'? Are Performance Appraisals a good use of your time? What architecture within our systems processes (4 of Spades) encourage you to perform at a high level?

We have this measure, you see, that so long as we are not incompetent, we are deemed competent. Which leaves a huge range of variability within which we can exist and not have to aim for any better.

I don't want you to work harder, because I know that ... you already work ... TOO HARD ...

(8 and 9 of Spades).

... when we compare what ... we do ... with what other people in other jobs do.

We want you to be able to work Smarter, Better, Safer. And in order to do that we all need to ... think more elegantly about how we do ... the things we do (4 of Spades again!)

"Doing what we do because that is the way we have always done it" (3 of Spades) is not an appropriate response in the emerging paradigm of the 'Science of Safety in Healthcare'.

We want more 'Flow', not more 'Woe'.

2 of Spades.

What does playing 'Words with Friends' or Facebook contribute to the care environment, and in particular what does it contribute to your working bandwidth when you care for your patient?

Let's have a talk about what situational awareness is, what it looks like ... and how we go about performing it.

We could even talk about whether we can maintain a high level of vigilance over the course of a full ten-hour day, and we can talk about where the opportunities and safety valves exist that allow us to be vigilant and be it well (9 of Spades).

Ace of Spades: Is hand hygiene STILL the most important thing you can do after all these years? And does the concept of five moments of hand hygiene translate well into our current recovery systems of work? (4 of Spades.)

King of Spades: When it comes to sorting out problems, do we stop thinking too soon? Do we stop our Root Cause Analysis as soon as we find someone to blame and yet still fret that within healthcare we still have a culture of blame?

Further, how would a simple technique such as mind-mapping help us discover more intelligent solutions when unfortunate circumstances implode because we drop imperfect people into imperfect systems and expect them to be prefect?

(Now that thought, right there, might just about involve every card in the deck!)

There may be some words you don't understand here: For example, 'Below Ten Thousand' and 'Shinobi', or even 'I'M SAFE'. But I can't leave you with NO Mysteries to solve, now can I? Where's the fun in that? It would be like exploring the Great Barrier Reef on Google Earth: "Sure, I've seen it, but I don't really feel like I've BEEN there!" It takes an immersion experience to do that!

This is profound stuff.

It's stuff we as professionals prefer not to think about. Let alone talk about, because it is challenging in a guttural sort of a way. But: It is an inevitable, and probably the most valuable part of the caring experience.

In actuality, it is, in totality, Standard 9 of the accreditation standards: 'Identification and Care of the Deteriorating Patient', except that in Recovery, we do it backwards. In Recovery, it is happily most often 'Identification and Care of the IMPROVING patient!'

(Because when patients come into our care, they are immediately as deteriorated as they are likely to get!)

In effect, it becomes a discussion on what you (and your manager) can do for yourselves (and each other) to potentiate the care environment ...

... how in the future you can use this information and these tools to manufacture a system whereby you can work safely and at a high level today, tomorrow, next month, next year, forever.

Because we are not employed by the hour. We're employed by the lifetime.

In order to provide for our students' continuing professional development, and because we can't teach them everything in the few opportunities that are available to us, we provide the READD outline online so that they can engage with it more fully at their own leisure and in their own time should they wish.

It's a prototype concept that is not quite complete as yet, but then again, what is?

A finishing point is only ever the starting point for something else.

(As I well know, because otherwise I wouldn't currently have an ant farm sitting on the breakfast bar at home ... but that's another story.)

So as you find gaps, and you will, I invite you to bridge them.

Equally important to the discussion of why things are there is the discussion of what should be there but isn't, and why and where you would include it if you wanted to.

So even if you don't agree with what we've done, you can still use it or use the template to create your own.

What we DON'T HAVE, for example, are: Wees, poos and spews. And if that's what interests you, that's what should be there.

What we DO HAVE, though, is a flexible, elastic, experiential starting point for engagement as well as a positive and strategic framework for inquisitive knowledge acquisition.

Shallow dive or dig deep. The choice is yours. As with all card tricks, most times ... The more you give, the more you get back.

So: what have we learned in the process?

Lesson 1:

Increasing engagement: All people, including students, have the desire to 'belong', to 'break into' a pre-existing group with uncertain group rules.

We have to be mindful of local organisational culture and pre-existing group dynamics.

We can apply ant-thropology here, but we aren't in the business of psychoanalysing people (or ants).

It's not that we're not qualified ... we just find it ... not very productive.

We just want to engage people in a supportive educational environment as best we can. And let the rest sort itself out as it will, and it can.

Lesson 2:

Employing Gamification: Gamification is more scientific than just 'making a game out of things'.

It is psychologically strategic and aims to deliver a purposeful outcome by engaging the brain on a completely different level to what we are traditionally used to.

It can be: fun challenging, with skills upgraded to just outside of your current reach (who wants a trophy?), to give a sense of accomplishment at each and every quantum step. (But you are going to have to earn it!)

It layers progression upon knowledge acquisition, so that knowledge evolves over the course of the journey (you get better at something) and it provides a rich interactive experience for the learner. (And you don't even realise it!)

In other words, for our students, it is something unique to remember the Recovery experience by, and thus hopefully, it becomes, for us, an opportunity to identify, and then hopefully attract, the best candidates back to us.

Lesson 3:

Exploring the Johari window:

The Johari window explores the boundaries of current and possible ranges of consciousness:

There are four panes to a Johari window, and this is my take on it:

- What you know you know
- What you know others know
- What you don't know you know
- And what you don't know you don't know

It gives us a metaphor to understand consciousness, both in ourselves and in the student.

It also helps us understand that: It doesn't matter that we don't always know. It helps students to know that we are happy to acknowledge our own fallibilities. And it gives us the opportunity to safely explore the unknown together.

Lesson 4:

Advancing planning through simulated simulations: Finally, READD doesn't have to be used just on students. READD provides an opportunity to challenge ourselves, at any given moment of any given day,

Because the card you hold could be the next challenge you receive.

Imagine a situation where the phenomenon on the card is being played out.

What do you do, what are the obstacles that get in the way of you doing what you want to do? And most important, what are the opportunities you can identify that would allow those things to be done better?

NOW we are into true learning territory, and for this, you will definitely need some Spades!

So, in conclusion, a deck of cards becomes an educational pathway.

I've tried to explain that to the ladies in the cafeteria where I buy my cards, but they seem to be having a bit of trouble getting their heads around the concept.

"Recovery quiet again, today?" they ask.

"Nope. Poker cards are an educational tool. They help us explore Standard 9 of the Accreditation Standards … but backwards!"

"Suuuuure!"

So. Are you READDy? Are you game? Pick a card! Any card!

Timelessness in the Desert

I first sensed timelessness in the Australian desert, somewhere about 300 km from Lake Eyre, the driest part of the Australian mainland.

The land was so old. It was almost as though time didn't exist, as if each moment was stretched out so far that it became imperceptible.

Being present in the moment became easy. All pretensions, distractions, extraneous thoughts, became nothing. There was nothing else you could do but just 'be'.

Some people might know it as mindfulness, being present in the moment.

But strings of mindfulness put together creates a timelessness that transforms a life.

In mindfulness we absorb ourselves in the moment. Absorbing ourselves in the moment, we perform our duty with focus.

An essential part of creating a monument to that moment is doing a good job.

Doing a good job means successful completion.

Part of successful completion is mopping up loose ends and tidying up afterwards.

The final sign-off cannot be complete without reflection. Reflection is learning. A team reflecting is a system learning.

If we are too busy to be mindful, too busy to be focused, too busy to mop up and tidy up, and too busy to reflect, then we are not privileging the doing of a good job.

And we are not interested in evolving our practice into systems learning.

We are only intent on surviving the day, no matter who we hurt in the process.

If your best practice doesn't exude timelessness in its nature, then the suffering you unwittingly create certainly will.

How can we be Authentic in healthcare, or in life, if we can't give ourselves the time we need to practise Authentically?

As clinicians we may be paid by the hour, but we are employed by the lifetime.

As clinical production unit entities we are owed synergy in work processes, and sustainability in work expectations, in order to maintain the stamina required to perform with precision and Authenticity our social contract.

As living sentient beings we are owed a duty of care which includes a balance in all things, including but not limited to our caring responsibilities to ourselves and significant others, and we are owed a duty of care to provide us with the opportunity to fulfil our aspirational hierarchy of needs, that is, if we are to maintain the stamina required to live a well-considered life.

I've seen too many good clinicians come crashing down simply because too much has been expected of too few and a sacrificial node has collapsed from underneath them.

Failure is too hard a way to learn about the limits of sustainability. And such preventable experiential suffering is too harsh a way to learn about your own Authenticity.

Whilst we avoid dealing with the problem, there is only one thing we can say with fatalism each time we witness a clinician fall like an angel with broken wings: In the words of Ned Kelly, Australian bushranger, "Such is life. I guess I should have known it would come to this."

The biggest shame is that we work in a humanity profession which devalues our humanity.

Harry had a dream the other night.

He was a passenger on a flight. The plane was approaching the landing strip, but something was wrong. The landing strip was bad. So the pilot put down on a highway under construction nearby.

"Was this a good dream or a bad dream?" he asked me.

My opinion was that it was a great dream.

Because when the future seems blocked, fate provides an alternate pathway, one you would never have envisaged, made all the more interesting for its innovativeness.

I reminded him of Sully: "We'll be in the Hudson." And Flight QF32 and the mere existence of the opportunity of the Armstrong Spiral.

A pathway un-envisaged, a pathway to try for a better future. Or stay the same, stick with the decrepit runway and punish your luck.

Human Factors

The greatest opportunity in healthcare in the modern era is the incorporation of human factors into the caring environment.

It is an opportunity that arises now because our intelligence has come to the final realisation that our stubbornness will not get us better results.

And as simple as human factors are, it will still take the rest of Rob's working life, and more, to implant it into the psyche and muscle memory of the healthcare system.

It will be an interesting journey, and the team that forms around Rob will help him implement a much-needed change that will result in the turnaround of quality care delivery to be the safest ever in all the history of medicine.

A new era will emerge from Rob's work, an era where we can truly, for the first time ever, first do no harm.

Human factors will be healthcare's parachute, and it will take all the Authenticity on offer of nurses, anaesthetists, surgeons and pilots to teach it to us.

For patients it will mean millions of spared lives. For hospitals it will be cost-neutral. I will be ecstatically happy if *Below Ten Thousand* is still packed as the emergency reserve chute in the event of the need for a cut-away.

In a valley lost to time a windsock blows gently in the breeze. The sky is a deep sapphire blue. The foothills rise green to the west. The sea glints perfectly, a welcome haven from the heat. There is a drop zone down there somewhere. There is nothing left to do but let go. Drop. Free fall into the void. And rejoice like hell when you hear the pop, feel your fall brake and see your feet rise up beneath you.

Your chute has opened. You are safe. All that is left to do is drift on the breeze back down to a welcoming earth. To arrive safe and sound to a world that never quite looks the same,

And a beer that never quite tastes the same,

Simply because you have left something behind up there in the clouds, a part of you jettisoned with the tug of a ripcord way back there in the sunglint sky ...

... your fear.

Regenerating a Supportive Culture

As I walk down the paddock, it is easier to see where I haven't been, than it is to see where I have been.

That is, it is easier to see where there are weeds, because weeds command more attention than regenerative pasture.

But once you learn to see rejuvenation, it becomes clear to the eye that in most of the important pasture zones there is nothing else but high-quality pasture.

So, at the moment of writing, the cows that graze the alluvial country we live on have 68% of the land under the best nutrition I can offer them.

Rejuvenation takes time, and regenerative farming takes, not just a vision, but a psychological buffer that will withstand the rhetoric of traditional farmers and their traditional farming methods.

Likewise in healthcare.

If the goal is to enable advocacy, to rejuvenate the safety culture that allows the clinician to advocate, first on behalf of themselves and then on behalf of the patient, then what has to change is our ability to reimagine the future with respect to our Authenticity.

To be Authentic to our goal of patient care requires a vision where Authenticity is allowed to flourish.

It also requires a buffer that protects us from the rhetoric of the past.

As in farming, a regenerative safety culture is not claiming what has been lost, but rather what has been eroded by the raging waters of an uncaring economy which sees numbers, but not necessarily the full extent of the meaning encapsulated within those numbers.

Thus, a person with a clipboard can see a nurse making a bed and think: "That's a person making a bed."

What they will not see is the numerous other transactions that take place during that simple act, such as the observation of a bruise, the assessing of mobility, the reassurance of the patient who sees an opportunity to ask a question about their treatment, the checking of cognitive state, nutritional status and a host of other things, most of which not even the nurse is aware they are doing.

So to replace the nurse with a lesser trained person because making a bed is just making a bed leaves a considerable part of the data out of the equation, which is then lost forever.

What is lost to the equation is the vision, the values, the strategic direction and the operational virtues that lead you to a hereto unattainable destination:

'To provide the most effective safety culture you can sustainably provide.'

So in advocacy, there are two things missing:

1) Advocacy training;

And

2) The will to listen.

To advocate is a cultural prerogative if engagement in a safety culture is a mandatory part of working in a hospital.

Nurses may or may not have been effectively coached on advocating for the patient with regards to clinical matters, but they have not been trained, nor coached, to advocate on behalf of themselves.

The misfortune here is that advocating on behalf of yourself or your profession is a big part of advocating for your patient, and the biggest problem is that we have deferred that right to our nursing unions who then use it as a bargaining tool at the enterprise bargaining negotiation table.

Safety should NOT be bargained. It is a right and it is NOT for negotiation.

As clinicians, nurses and doctors, get better trained at advocacy, the next step is to create a culture that prioritises Listening Skills.

Because at the end of the day, it is the will to listen from which follows a will to act.

Only once you have the skills, and the will, to listen, will you then have the ghost of a chance at effective action.

The skills benefit us in all directions.

A lot of farming is about listening. Listening to the seasons, the animals, the pasture in order to understand their needs and their possibilities.

Once you accept your assigned duty of care, not to listen is a form of brutality, a brutality simply because the harm that flows from such ignorance is unnecessary.

Farmers are no less immune to thinking errors than health professionals. We often think that farming is about growing animals and crops to cash in at market. But farming, in reality, is about growing people. Families. The economic pursuit is simply a means of production. To listen is to understand. It helps us from focusing on the wrong thing.

When Joanne Hughes tried to advocate on behalf of her little 'cheeky' daughter, Jasmine, it was the others' will to listen that let her down with catastrophic consequences.

A person trained to advocate is also a person trained to listen, and so the perils of oppositional defiance, thinking errors, cognitive bias and the groupthink of positional power all dissipate, if not entirely (because we *are* only human), then at least hopefully sufficiently for our 'will to act' to have a chance.

In organisations as big as healthcare institutions invariably are, what does it take to make someone listen?

In advocating on behalf of colleagues in the past, there have been a few useful parameters which have informed our strategies to achieve a logical outcome.

The first is to acknowledge a *vision*.

Hospital values, safety, and the desire to strive for a just culture are a good place to start.

The second is to acknowledge the *parameters* within which to conduct the discussion.

Legislation, policies, procedures, Standards and guidelines all form the parameters from within which the outcome should be considered.

The third step is to acknowledge the default *baseline*, that is, the bottom level the performance, resource and ethical limits impose on us which constitutes the line we must defend.

From there, the *evidence*, such as there is, should be acknowledged and its validity established.

If the evidence supports the need to act, then all that is left is to make the decision to act.

How you shall act is a matter for latter discussion and contemplation, because the answers to the conundrum may not yet be apparent.

If a strategy and a framework for progression is agreed on, then the action performed can be monitored, with feedback loops instilled at every point to assess for sequential improvement or corruptive processes at every level.

In the end, what would such a thing look like?

It looks like Authenticity.

And out of Authenticity comes the reality of a better future.

A future where Jasmine lives!

If you have made it this far, you are truly awesome and we all want you as our nurse.

I hope you have a brilliant career, a brilliant life, and may your loved ones, the ones you most cherish in those private moments you call your own be glad they have, at the centre of their world an Authentic nurse who cares for themselves simply so that they can care fully for others in the midst of a life well lived.

Good luck!

Pete!

Exam question

"Safety is a Trojan horse that steals into our healthcare realm rather than the walls that keep us safe."

(Pete Smith, 2021)

Can Authenticity help?
Discuss.

(1000 word limit)

About the Author

Pete Smith is just a guy at the shallow end of the gene pool. He spent the first five years of his life under a farmhouse playing in the dirt with his Matchbox® cars.

He spent the next eleven years surrounded by cows.

His brother, Greg, five years older, had severe Down Syndrome. Greg was much, much cooler than Pete could ever be.

So how did this kid who knew more about cows than humans end up as a career nurse? And how did this unpolished introvert finish up philosophising on nursing?

The world is a mysterious place. Some would say complex, dangerous and chaotic.

But really, it is quite simple if we allow it to be.

When he is not doing farming stuff, drinking coffee with his awe-inspiring wife or chopping Granny's wood, he may be found in his Cognitive Laboratory conversing with his totally awesome international collaborators and constructing mind maps on whiteboards.

Pete's motto?

"I think, therefore I ... ummm?"

www.ingramcontent.com/pod-product-compliance
Ingram Content Group UK Ltd.
Pitfield, Milton Keynes, MK11 3LW, UK
UKHW022210230426
12048UKWH00016BA/757